THIRD EDITION

Communication
for Nurses

TALKING WITH PATIENTS

Edited by

Lisa Kennedy Sheldon, PhD, APRN-BC, AOCNP®

Assistant Professor
University of Massachusetts, Boston
Boston, Massachusetts

Oncology Nurse Practitioner
St. Joseph Hospital
Nashua, New Hampshire

Associate Member
Dana-Farber/Harvard Cancer Centers

Janice B. Foust, PhD, RN
Assistant Professor
University of Massachusetts, Boston
Boston, Massachusetts

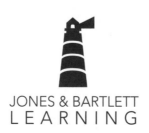

JONES & BARTLETT
L E A R N I N G

3-6-14
GB
$60.95

World Headquarters
Jones & Bartlett Learning
5 Wall Street
Burlington, MA 01803
978-443-5000
info@jblearning.com
www.jblearning.com

Jones & Bartlett Learning books and products are available through most bookstores and online booksellers. To contact Jones & Bartlett Learning directly, call 800-832-0034, fax 978-443-8000, or visit our website, www.jblearning.com.

Substantial discounts on bulk quantities of Jones & Bartlett Learning publications are available to corporations, professional associations, and other qualified organizations. For details and specific discount information, contact the special sales department at Jones & Bartlett Learning via the above contact information or send an email to specialsales@jblearning.com.

Production Credits

Executive Publisher: William Brottmiller
Senior Editor: Amanda Harvey
Editorial Assistant: Rebecca Myrick
Production Editor: Keith Henry
Senior Marketing Manager: Jennifer Stiles
V.P., Manufacturing and Inventory Control: Therese Connell
Composition: diacriTech
Rights & Photo Research Coordinator: Joseph Veiga

Cover Design: Scott Moden
Cover Images: Nurse in red with man in wheelchair © Monkey Business Images/ShutterStock, Inc.; Nurse in light purple with woman in bed © Monkey Business Images/ShutterStock, Inc.; Male nurse with young boy © Wavebreak Media/Thinkstock
Printing and Binding: Edwards Brothers Malloy
Cover Printing: Edwards Brothers Malloy

Library of Congress Cataloging-in-Publication Data
Kennedy-Sheldon, Lisa, author.
  Communication for nurses : talking with patients / Lisa Kennedy Sheldon, Janice B. Foust.—Third edition.
    p. ; cm.
  Includes bibliographical references and index.
  ISBN 978-1-4496-9177-6 (pbk.)
  I. Foust, Janice B., author. II. Title.
  [DNLM: 1. Nurse-Patient Relations. 2. Communication. 3. Models, Nursing. 4. Nurses—psychology. 5. Nursing Theory. WY 88]
  RT23
  610.7306'99—dc23
                                                                    2013022672

6048
Printed in the United States of America
17 16 15 14 13   10 9 8 7 6 5 4 3 2 1

DEDICATION

To my parents ... from my first words

—Lisa Kennedy Sheldon

To future nurses and colleagues

—Janice B. Foust

TABLE OF CONTENTS

SECTION II　　THE NURSE–PATIENT RELATIONSHIP

SECTION IV   DIFFICULT COMMUNICATION

SECTION V COMMUNICATING WITH OTHER HEALTHCARE PROVIDERS

SECTION VI CONCLUSION

ACKNOWLEDGMENTS

No publication is a solo effort, and particularly not one about communication. Many of my friends, family members, and colleagues have listened to my ideas about improving communication in health care.

First, I want to thank all the people who have allowed me to participate in their health care over the years. Your stories have inspired me and profoundly changed my life, both professionally and personally. My ability to talk with my patients has changed and continues to evolve because of each of you. I am humbled by your trust and truly honored to be a part of your care.

To my colleagues at the University of Massachusetts, Boston and St. Joseph Hospital, I appreciate your patience, wisdom, and wonderful—often humorous—contributions to this text. To the staff at Jones & Bartlett Learning, I appreciate all your efforts on behalf of this text.

Finally, I want to acknowledge my family—my parents, Everett (Ray) and Louise Kennedy; Meredith, Laurie, and Everett Kennedy; Zane Shatzer; Jay Gardner; Paul, Grace, Jamie, Judy, Patty, and Margaret Sheldon—for talking, listening, laughing, and sharing your lives with me. To my children—Brad, Greg, Andrea, and Luke—thank you for all the joy and endless light you bring to my life. And, finally, to my husband, Tom, I want to express my love and gratitude for your ongoing support—you are my foundation.

—Lisa Kennedy Sheldon

I am so grateful to my wonderful family—past and present—as well as my many friends and colleagues who have supported, encouraged, and inspired me, both during my early formative years before I became a nurse and then continuing throughout my career. To my family, special thanks for sharing your lives, laughter, encouragement, and love.

As a nurse, I am grateful to the numerous patients and their families who have shared their amazing stories and experiences. I am impressed by how you faced difficult situations with grace, and in doing so, you helped me become a better nurse.

To all my wonderful colleagues and mentors, too numerous to mention individually, I thank you. From you, I learned to value the importance of collaboration and exemplary communication skills as ways to improve patient care by working together and bringing out the best in teams. Your leadership, passion, and drive to improve the rigor and visibility of nursing practice continue to motivate me. I also want to thank the Jones & Bartlett Learning staff for all their help in the making of this text.

—Janice B. Foust

ABOUT THE AUTHORS

Lisa Kennedy Sheldon, PhD, APRN, is on the faculty at the University of Massachusetts, Boston, is a writer and researcher, and works as an oncology nurse practitioner at St. Joseph Hospital in Nashua, New Hampshire. She graduated from Saint Anselm College with a bachelor of science degree in nursing. After working in a variety of oncology settings, Dr. Sheldon attended Boston College, where she obtained a master of science degree in nursing as an oncology clinical nurse specialist. Later, she returned to Boston College to obtain postgraduate certification as a nurse practitioner. Dr. Sheldon holds a doctor of philosophy degree from the College of Nursing at the University of Utah with a concentration in cancer control and research. Dr. Sheldon's postdoctoral fellowship was at the Dana-Farber Cancer Institute's Cantor Center with her mentor and research collaborator, Donna L. Berry, PhD, RN, AOCN, FAAN.

Dr. Sheldon has published several books, book chapters, and articles, and has served as an associate editor for the *Clinical Journal of Oncology Nursing*. She serves on national and international panels and advisory boards and is the co-director of the Global Nursing Caucus. She delivers educational programs to healthcare providers and community groups, and presents nationally and internationally on cancer nursing, oncology care, and communication research. Dr. Sheldon's program of research focuses on patient–provider communication, oncology nursing, and issues in global cancer care.

Janice B. Foust, PhD, RN, is an Assistant Professor at the University of Massachusetts, Boston, College of Nursing and Health Sciences. After graduating from the University of New Hampshire with a bachelor of science degree in nursing, she later obtained a master of science degree in nursing from Boston College as a clinical nurse specialist. She earned her doctor of philosophy degree from the University of Pennsylvania, School of Nursing, where she also completed her postdoctoral training as a Claire M. Fagin Fellow in the John A. Hartford Foundation, *Building Academic Nursing Capacity* program, guided by her mentor, Mary D. Naylor, PhD, FAAN, RN.

Dr. Foust's program of research focuses on care transitions of older adults, and more specifically on the issues of posthospital medication management. She has published several articles and book chapters, along with presenting her work at local, regional, and national conferences. Dr. Foust has also served as manuscript reviewer for national and international journals. She has held clinical, research, and leadership positions within various practice settings, such as home health care and academic teaching hospitals.

PREFACE

■ CASE STUDY

A 42-year-old man comes to the oncology center to begin chemotherapy for metastatic renal cell carcinoma. The chart says his first name is Edmund, and the staff begins calling him Ed. He is a quiet man and often does not share much with the nurses during his weekly chemotherapy. One day, 3 months into his treatment, the nurse looks at his chart to assess his status prior to beginning chemotherapy. She says, "Ed, I was just looking at your chart and thinking Edmund must be a family name. What do you like to be called?" The patient answered, "Mike. I never liked my first name."

■ OVERVIEW

How embarrassing! The staff assumed that he must be called Ed. It would have taken only a moment during the first visit to discover his preferences.

Small mistakes take place every day between nurses and patients. Some are based on assumptions, such as calling the patient by the wrong name, and others may be more complicated, such as not understanding a patient's pain because of cultural differences in the expression of pain. As nurses, we do not intentionally misunderstand our patients, nor do we want to hurt them. It takes a few minutes a day to not only improve how well we talk with our patients, but also how well we listen to what they are telling us. Better understanding of patients' experiences, preferences, and resources improves the ability of both nurses and patients to set more realistic goals and plan more appropriate interventions.

Becoming better communicators means changing our ability to relate to people who happen to be our patients. I want to compare your communication skills to a geographical situation. In Japan, there is a beautiful mountain called Mount Fuji. Not only is this peak picturesque, but it is also where three of the earth's tectonic plates meet and collide. The pressures in the earth related to these plates have caused frequent tremors and even deadly earthquakes. To combat the dangerous consequences of tremors, many Japanese buildings have been seismically retrofitted not only to be functional, but also to withstand the earth's shaking. Some buildings have deep pilings that secure them to bedrock and prevent collapse. Others have sliding plates between the foundation and the upper stories of the building to allow the building to slide during seismic activity.

Like these buildings, your communication skills may be functional, even admirable, but they need to be able to withstand the forces that will challenge them every day. Perhaps a deeper understanding of your values or more flexibility in discussing sensitive issues will enhance your ability to listen and respond to your patients. The goal of this text is to develop your communication skills by providing a sturdy foundation and introducing techniques that will withstand the stressful healthcare environment to help you become a better communicator. Along the way, you will learn about your professional and moral obligations, your own values and personality, and the resources available to provide a foundation for your clinical interactions with patients.

■ HOW THIS TEXT IS STRUCTURED

Many of the techniques discussed in this text are meant to enhance professional and personal development. The text first takes a closer look at patients and nurses as people and at ethical, legal, and professional guidelines for communication as a facet of nursing care. A detailed chapter reviews the therapeutic relationship from the beginning through the actual provision of nursing care and, finally, to the closure of the relationship. Interviewing skills are reviewed as both a science and an art, with case studies serving as examples of potential clinical encounters.

Next, the text examines communication with specific patient populations and situations. How do you deal with a patient in a crisis situation? How do you communicate with an intubated patient? What is the best way to give constructive criticism to a colleague? These are a few of the topics covered here as part of practical approaches to difficult communication situations. They are intended to serve as guidelines for when you are at a loss for words.

Finally, in response to requests and changes within the profession, the third edition of this text contains new sections on compassion and the emotional work of nursing, the nature of suffering, and working with colleagues. Additionally, websites have been added to provide more extensive online resources, and the references have been updated.

With time and experience, you will grow into the nurse and communicator you want to be, given your personal strengths and professional goals. A nurse may be respectful, caring, funny, sensitive, insightful, precise, concise, empathetic, spiritual, inquisitive, logical, gentle, and peaceful. Each nurse is a unique mixture of many qualities. The development of your communication style is up to you.

CONTRIBUTORS

Teri Aronowitz, PhD, FNP-BC
University of Massachusetts, Boston
College of Nursing and Health Sciences
Boston, Massachusetts

Jeannie M. Brant, PhD, APRN, AOCN
Billings Clinic
Montana State University
Billings, Montana

Sheryl LaCoursiere, PhD, FNP-BC, APRN
University of Massachusetts, Boston
College of Nursing and Health Sciences
Yale University
New Haven, Connecticut

JoAnn Mulready-Shick, EdD, RN, CNE, ANEF
University of Massachusetts, Boston
College of Nursing and Health Sciences
Boston, Massachusetts

Amy Rex-Smith, DNSc, RN, ACNS, BC
University of Massachusetts, Boston
College of Nursing and Health Sciences
Boston, Massachusetts

Esther Seibold, DNSc, RN
University of Massachusetts, Boston
College of Nursing and Health Sciences
Boston, Massachusetts

Jennifer Mardin Small, RN, MSN
University of Massachusetts, Boston
College of Nursing and Health Sciences
Boston, Massachusetts

Judith Healey Walsh, EdD(c), MS, RN
University of Massachusetts, Boston
College of Nursing and Health Sciences
Boston, Massachusetts

Setting the Stage for Effective Communication

CHAPTER ONE

The First Encounter

Lisa Kennedy Sheldon

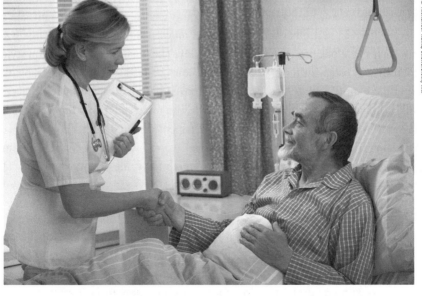

■ CASE STUDY

"Good Morning, Mrs. T. My name is Jay, and I will be your nurse today. We have a full day today with some tests. How about getting washed up now? Is it all right to call you Mrs. T.?"

Mrs. T. is a 76-year-old woman with metastatic lung cancer being cared for by the nurse, Jay. It is her second day in the hospital after developing a fever and cough. She is quiet, giving one-word answers to Jay's questions. Mrs. T. thinks that Jay is being too aggressive, making her wash up and scheduling tests without asking her permission. Jay is beginning to wonder about why Mrs. T. is reluctant to talk with him.

Later, when he comes in to bring her morning medications, Jay says, "Mrs. T., I have your medications." She responds, "What am I supposed to do, take those now just because you say so?"

Introduction

In each room, bed, or chair, nurses encounter different people seeking health care. Each time a nurse meets a new person in a healthcare setting, a new relationship begins for both parties. These relationships often develop at vulnerable points, when people seek assessment, treatment, information, and often reassurance about their health. Some interactions will proceed smoothly, with both parties having the same goals for the visit. At other times, the nurse may encounter more challenging situations, such as the one presented in the case study. The nurse's communication style and responses will establish the framework for future conversations and the implementation of the plan of care. Often, it is the unspoken communication that influences the words to follow. The nurse's role is to explore and understand both the patient's needs and the healthcare goals in order to deliver patient-centered care. High-quality communication in health care requires more than words; it requires careful tailoring of communication for the interaction and, most importantly, the person who is the patient.

Terminology

For the purposes of this text, it is useful to define the terms used for the people involved in communication in the healthcare setting. *Patients* are people seeking and/or receiving healthcare services from healthcare providers. While the term "clients" is sometimes used in nursing and communication literature, the term "patients" will be used in this text because it conveys a level of ethical responsibility to a person in a vulnerable position seeking services.

Healthcare providers are sometimes described in books as "clinicians" or by healthcare profession, such as "doctors" or "nurses." This text discusses just one type of healthcare provider—nurses.

Patient–provider communication refers to the communication between the patient, family member(s), and provider(s) during visits to receive health care, often involving multiple types of healthcare providers. Much of patient–provider communication is similar across healthcare professions, and improving communication requires an interdisciplinary approach.

The *nurse–patient relationship* is a different type of relationship, as it involves the nurse as a professional healthcare provider communicating with a person seeking health care. Gone are many of the social boundaries that define everyday relationships. Both parties have expectations about how the interaction will proceed and what the outcomes will be. These are different relationships—ones that have the potential to affect both patients and nurses. Communication is a process of mutual influence.

During healthcare visits, patients are often placed in dependent, vulnerable roles. Within a short period of time, they may be required to reveal intimate information about their lives and bodies to people (healthcare providers) they have just met, or they may even undergo painful procedures. For patients to feel respected, cared for, and safe, nurses must create an environment that puts patients at ease, allowing revelation, understanding, and mutual planning to facilitate assessment, treatment, and healing or perhaps peaceful death.

Health care is a fast-paced environment. Time is often short, and quickly establishing these relationships may sound like an impossible task. Nevertheless, good communication is a clinical skill that can be learned. Beginning with basic education, nurses learn the fundamentals of establishing the relationship, basic communication skills, and specific nursing interventions. These professional skills build on previous experiences and begin a lifetime of learning for the professional nurse as both a person and a communicator. After graduation, nurses use their clinical experiences with patients and families to build and refine their own communication style. Each room, chair, and bed brings a unique situation requiring nurses to become flexible communicators.

Communication is a universal word with many meanings. It has been described as a transfer of information between a message sender and a message receiver. In nursing, communication entails a sharing of health-related information between a patient and a nurse, with both participants acting as senders and receivers of information. Communication occurs in many ways and may be verbal or nonverbal, written or spoken, culturally appropriate, personal or impersonal, issue specific, or even relationship oriented. It can pertain in a larger sense to public health campaigns and policy issues, or to information on the Internet, or to a single patient's personal experience with a health issue. Human communication is a continuous and dynamic process, with the nurse and patient developing a relationship not only to share information but also to facilitate health, growth, and healing.

Theoretical Background

Human communication is multidimensional and has been studied by researchers from many disciplines, including nursing, medicine, psychology, social work, and pastoral care. Watzlawick, Beavin, and Jackson (1967) describe communication as occurring on two levels: the relationship level and the content level. The relationship level refers to how the two participants are bound to each other. The content level refers to the words, language, and information that are exchanged by the participants. The two levels are inextricably bound, and the content is relayed more effectively in healthy relationships. The opposite occurs in strained relationships—that is, the content of the message is not clearly relayed or heard because of struggles within the relationship.

Relationships between patients and healthcare providers such as nurses influence communication and care. This section reviews four models of communication with applicability to nurse–patient communication in the healthcare setting. While not distinctly nursing theories, each contributes to the understanding and provides theoretical frameworks for communication models and some components of nursing theory (see the chapter titled *The Nurse as a Person: Theories of Self and Nursing* for more on nursing theories). The models to be discussed are as follows:

- Health Belief Model
- Orlando's theory of the deliberative nursing process
- Rogerian model
- Social information processing models

The Health Belief Model

The Health Belief Model (Rosenstock, 1974) focuses on the patient's perspective on health communication. This model has been influential because it explains how the patient's beliefs may predict the adoption of healthy behaviors. Certain variables or modifying factors can influence a patient's beliefs, including demographic characteristics such as age, sex, and ethnicity; perceived threats; and cues to action (e.g., advice, advertising, or illness in a family member). When applying the Health Belief Model, cues to action are incorporated into interventions to optimize their effectiveness in changing behaviors. For example, young adolescents are more susceptible to cigarette advertisements (*cues to action*) and peer pressure (*age-related variable*) than are middle-aged adults. Therefore, advertising campaigns to stop adolescents from smoking may be more effective if they involve posting videos of students placing body bags in front of the corporate headquarters of tobacco companies on YouTube rather than providing handouts for parents at the pediatrician's office. In contrast, a diagnosis of lung cancer in a family member (*cue to action*) would be more apt to influence a middle-aged adult to quit smoking than it would a teenager. Communication at the nurse–patient level should be geared toward understanding patients' perceptions of their health and utilizing interventions that are appropriate for their demographic characteristics.

Orlando's Theory of the Deliberative Nursing Process

Nursing communication affects patient outcomes such as anxiety, adherence to treatments, and satisfaction with care. Ida Jean Orlando's theory of nursing process describes nurses' reactions to patients' behavior as generating a perception, thought, and feeling in the nurse and then action by the nurse.

Orlando's theory of the deliberative nursing process describes communication between nurses and patients in terms of three concepts: the "patient's behavior," the "nurse's reaction," and the "nurse's activity." The patient sends a cue in the form of a behavior—that is, "patient's behavior." The "nurse's reaction" is the nurse's response to the "patient's behavior." Two types of nurse responses are defined in Orlando's theory: a "nonobservable response" consisting of a thought, perception, and feeling, and an observable "nurse's activity" as the final action/response to the "patient's behavior." Orlando further described the "nurse's activity" as being "automatic" or "deliberative nursing process." The "deliberative nursing process" allows nurses to identify the patient's needs and help the patient—that is, to be of

Nurses develop communication skills that build on a lifetime of experience and continue to grow throughout their professional careers.

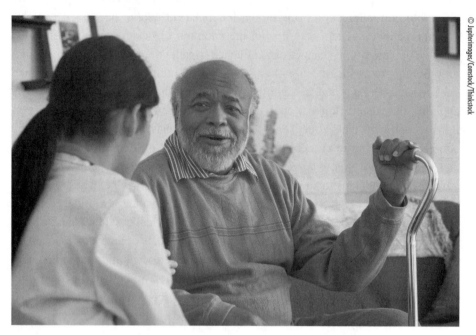

© Jupiterimages/Comstock/Thinkstock

help. Orlando's theory emphasizes that effective nursing practice is the result of the nurse's nonobservable reaction (perception, thought, and/or feeling), followed by the nurse's observable actions (activity) to the "patient's behavior."

In Orlando's theory, nurse–patient interaction involves reciprocity, making the relationship dynamic and collaborative. According to Orlando, the nurse confirms his or her perception, thought, and feeling with the patient for validation prior to selecting the activity. Deliberative actions are seen as more effective, but the process of self-reflection, the assessment of self-efficacy, and the role of peer evaluation/support are not clearly identified in the theory.

Rogerian Model

The Rogerian model describes the role of the relationship between the healthcare provider and the client or patient. Carl Rogers (1951) described the therapeutic relationship as central to facilitating healthy adjustment in the client. Communication is client centered because the patient is the focus of the interactions. The helper or healthcare provider communicates with empathy, positive regard (or respect), and congruence (or genuineness) to facilitate client adjustment to the circumstances and movement toward health. Although originally created for psychotherapists, the Rogerian model has proved useful for nursing and the establishment of the therapeutic nurse–patient relationship.

Model of Social Information Processing

Models of social information processing provide useful constructs that are applicable to how nurses learn to respond to patients. The Crick and Dodge model (Crick & Dodge, 1994) is a circular depiction of the emotional and cognitive processes involved in learning to respond to social cues. At the core of the model is a database of memories, acquired social rules, and social knowledge and schemas. When applied to nursing, this database may include previous social experiences in the personal and professional spheres, formal education in communication skills, and role expectations, including ethical and legal ramifications, societal expectations, and professional mandates of nursing. Nurses learn to develop their professional communication skills by regulating arousal (i.e., nurses controlling their internal reactions to patient communication, particularly during difficult conversations), developing self-efficacy (confidence), deciding on responses, and finally enacting a response that helps both patient and nurse attain their goals. Nurses adapt to their roles as professional healthcare providers by learning effective methods of responding to patients and developing confidence to communicate confidently in a variety of patient situations.

Summary

Communication is the sharing of information between individuals. It is also a dynamic and reciprocal process, affecting each person in the relationship. The communication process is influenced by the information to be shared and the structure of the relationship.

In health care, theoretical frameworks provide a basis for understanding nurse–patient communication. The Health Belief Model is useful in understanding why patients adopt or change health behaviors. Orlando's theory describes the nursing process in terms of nurses' reactions to patients' behaviors as generating a perception, thought, and feeling in the nurse and then action by the nurse. The communication is influenced by perceptions and judgments made by both the patient and the nurse (Sheldon & Ellington, 2008). The Rogerian model describes a patient-centered model for nurse–patient relationships. In this model, nurses use empathy, congruence, and positive regard/respect to establish a therapeutic relationship with the patient. Social information processing models provide useful constructs for exploring how nurses learn to respond to patients, including regulation of their internal reactions. These selected models demonstrate the dynamic process of healthcare communication and the fundamental components of nurse–patient communication.

Case Study Resolution

In the case study, Mrs. T. has certain perceptions about the nurse, Jay, and his role as her nurse. Jay is unsure about her reactions when he discussed her scheduled testing and morning care. Using a Rogerian approach, the nurse could explore Mrs. T.'s perceptions of the situation and offer suggestions about ways to incorporate her goals into the plan of care. What should have been a beginning to their relationship has become more challenging because certain parts of messages are missing, and the relationship is not well established. Perhaps Jay could respond, "Mrs. T., it can be difficult to be a patient. You haven't had much time to yourself since we scheduled these tests." Or perhaps he could give her more control over her day: "When would you like me to bring your medicine?" He could also acknowledge her underlying concerns: "You sound upset this morning. Tell me more about what's going on."

Whatever approach Jay takes is essential to establishing goals that are respectful of the patient and acknowledge her concerns regarding this experience. The lack of understanding on both sides can be minimized by effective communication and will lay the foundation for future interactions and optimal nursing care.

EXERCISES

Break into groups of three. Each person in the group has a role: a nurse, a patient, or an observer. Each person in the group will role-play in one role for 5 minutes. Pick one of the following scenarios:

- A 17-year-old boy with a seizure disorder who is not taking his medications regularly
- A 49-year-old man with a 2-pack-a-day smoking habit for 35 years who has bronchitis

- A 20-year-old woman with a chlamydial infection and a new sexual partner
- A 77-year-old woman with a recent transient ischemic attack and dizziness who does not like using a cane
- A 7-year-old boy who broke his wrist skateboarding and was not wearing protective gear

Begin the role-play with a greeting from the nurse and the initial assessment. Role-play for no more than 5 minutes. As the "nurse," begin the encounter with the appropriate introductions and assess the reason the "patient" has sought health care. As the "nurse," try to assess the "patient's" problem and arrive at mutually set goals. The "observer" will assess the "nurse's" actions.

After each role-play, the observer will begin the discussion with the group. Use the following questions to assess the interactions:

1. Did the nurse begin the relationship in a warm, respectful manner?

2. Did the nurse solicit the patient's perception of the situation?

3. Did the nurse make judgments about the patient's behavior?

4. Was the nurse empathetic to the patient's feelings about the situation?

5. Did the nurse ask the patient's opinion about possible interventions?

6. Did the nurse incorporate the patient's health beliefs into the plan of care?

Rotate the roles and pick a new patient scenario two more times so each person in the group has the opportunity to role-play each role.

References

Crick, N. R., & Dodge, K. A. (1994). A review and reformulation of social-information-processing mechanisms in children's social adjustment. *Psychological Bulletin, 1*(15), 74–101.

Rogers, C. (1951). *Client-centered therapy: Its practice, implications and theory.* London: Constable.

Rosenstock, I. M. (1974). The Health Belief Model and preventive health behavior. *Health Education Monographs, 2,* 354–386.

Sheldon, L. K., & Ellington, L. (2008). Application of a model of social information processing to nursing theory: How nurses respond to patients. *Journal of Advanced Nursing,* 388–398.

Watzlawick, P., Beavin, J., & Jackson, D. D. (1967). *Pragmatics of human communication.* New York: Norton.

CHAPTER TWO

The Nurse as a Person: Theories of Self and Nursing

Lisa Kennedy Sheldon

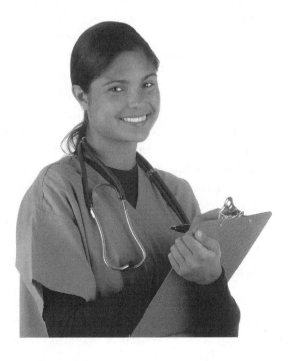

■ CASE STUDY

Susan is a 21-year-old senior in nursing school. She has always wanted to be a nurse but is having difficulty during her current clinical rotation in pediatrics. For the past two clinical days, she has been assigned to work with Alyssa, a 4-year-old child with acute lymphocytic leukemia (ALL). While undergoing maintenance chemotherapy, Alyssa developed neutropenia and a fever of unknown origin, requiring hospitalization for intravenous antibiotics. Today, Susan is changing Alyssa's pajamas after her morning bath. She looks at the little girl: bald from chemotherapy, pale and limp from anemia and infection. Unexpectedly, Susan finds herself starting to cry. Alyssa sees her eyes begin to fill with tears and asks Susan, "What's wrong? Are you hurt?"

Introduction

Nurses, like all human beings, are complex organisms with feelings, fears, hopes, and needs. Like other humans, nurses are the product of their genetic makeup, family environment, peer networks, cultural background, and previous experiences. Becoming an effective nurse requires identifying the characteristics that make each person unique, including oneself. The process of self-examination requires a more personal and honest reflection about the effect of past and present influences on current behavior. Most nursing students want to develop into kind, respectful, and effective professionals. They are motivated to understand and work with their patients to promote comfort, understanding, and healing in a patient-centered manner. However, to become a successful nurse requires understanding the wide variety of human responses to stressful circumstances in the healthcare setting. Students need to develop into nurses who use the knowledge and skills of nursing in a manner that allows for accurate assessments, mutual goal setting, and timely interventions that address patient needs. Understanding human responses—both the nurse's and the patients'—requires knowledge of the self.

Self-Awareness

The terms *self, self-concept, known self,* and *self-awareness* are frequently used in human developmental theories. The *self* is a personal definition of oneself that is distinct from other people. The *self-concept* is the judgments and attitudes about the self; it explains behavior and provides a framework for decision making. The *known self* comprises that part of the self that is consciously acknowledged. When choices are made within the context of the known self, then self-identity and self-worth are affirmed. *Self-awareness* is the active process of learning about the components of the self.

In nursing, understanding the self facilitates therapeutic interactions with patients. Because nurses often advocate for patients in healthcare systems, they need to distinguish between what are patients' experiences and what may be nurses' reactions. Accurate assessment and interventions require separating patients' experiences from the nurses' reactions. If nurses can separate their personal reactions from the patients' needs, then communication is more patient centered. While this may sound obvious and simple, it takes years of clinical experience to fully develop this ability. A deeper understanding of the self promotes growth in the nurse personally while enhancing professional communication with patients.

Theoretical Background

Many theorists have tried to explain the origins of the self. Harry Stack Sullivan (1892–1949) wrote extensively on how the self develops, and he developed a theory of interpersonal relations. Sullivan, an American psychoanalyst, believed that the self or self-system emerges during infancy as the result of an interpersonal relationship with a significant other (Sullivan, 1953). He identified two prime motivating factors for behavior: the need for satisfaction and the need for security. During the first year of life, if the basic needs for food, water, warmth, and tenderness are met, then the infant feels secure and satisfied. Conversely, if certain basic needs are not met, then tensions, such as anxiety and fear, develop in the child. A lack of security during childhood can produce anxiety that later stifles the development of healthy relationships in the adult. On the professional level, Sullivan described the therapeutic relationship as a healing, human connection between the provider and the patient.

The nursing theorist Hildegard Peplau built on Sullivan's theories, applying them to nursing practice. In her theory of interpersonal relations, Peplau described the phases of the interpersonal process that occur when a nurse and a patient come together during a health-related difficulty (Fawcett & Desanto-Madeya, 2012). Peplau defined nursing as a significant, therapeutic, and interpersonal process that functions cooperatively with other human processes to make health possible. She was the first to develop an interpersonal model of nursing practice, moving away from what nurses do *to* patients and toward what nurses do *with* patients. Nursing, as an interaction phenomenon, is not just a process of observation and intervention, but rather an active engagement of nurses with their patients. Peplau (1992) also described the *nurse-as-person* as significantly influencing patient outcomes and quality of life. According to Peplau, nurses function within six roles:

1. Stranger role: The nurse receives the patient as a stranger, providing a climate that promotes trust.
2. Resource role: The nurse gives information, answers questions, and interprets clinical information.
3. Teaching role: The nurse serves as teacher to the learner/patient, giving instruction and training.
4. Counseling role: The nurse provides guidance and encouragement to help the patient integrate his or her current life experience.
5. Surrogate role: The nurse works on the patient's behalf and helps the patient clarify domains of independence, dependence, and interdependence.
6. Active leadership role: The nurse assists the patient in achieving responsibility for treatment goals in a mutually satisfying way.

Peplau (1992) further developed her theory by describing the nurse–patient relationship as a dynamic process that creates the opportunity for learning and growth for both the patient and the nurse. This working relationship has three phases, as described by Peplau:

- Orientation phase
- Working phase
- Resolution/termination phase

During the *orientation phase*, the nurse and patient meet each other as strangers and develop a working partnership to address the health concerns of the patient. The nurse also performs an assessment of the patient's needs.

The *working phase* has two components: identification and exploitation. The identification component is when the nurse and the patient clarify ideas and expectations for the relationship and the nurse develops a nursing care plan. During the exploitation part of the working phase, the nurse helps the patient identify healthcare services and personal resources and implement strategies to resolve the health issues.

During the *resolution/termination phase*, the nurse and the patient evaluate the current health status. The nurse also makes referrals, as necessary, to continue care beyond the relationship. (See the *Establishing a Therapeutic Relationship* chapter for further exploration of the nurse–patient relationship.)

Theorists from other disciplines expanded the understanding of interpersonal communication. Sigmund Freud (1937), for example, provided well-known insights into human behavior. Freud is famous for his descriptions of the id, ego, and superego, but he also developed the ideas of transference and countertransference. *Transference* is the projection of one's attitudes or feelings from the past onto people in the present. For example, a female patient who is nervous about an upcoming surgery might say, "My husband hates hospitals." *Countertransference* refers to feelings that a nurse may develop about a patient's behaviors that have their roots in the nurse's previous life experiences. For example, suppose a nurse is caring for a male patient who is angry about being hospitalized. Perhaps the nurse avoids caring for the patient because of negative experiences with an angry male member of his own family. Recognizing feelings of countertransference helps nurses acknowledge their own feelings and allows a more objective reaction to patients' responses. Often, sharing these confusing feelings with trusted colleagues or mentors can help nurses gain more perspective about personality traits that inhibit responses or provoke negative or prejudiced judgments about patients.

Freud also identified *ego defense mechanisms* as other components of personality. These mechanisms allow people to protect themselves during anxiety-producing situations; examples include denial, projection, and rationalization. *Denial* is the lack of acceptance of a proven condition. For example, a mother whose child has leukemia might not be able to say that her child has cancer, but she can acknowledge that her child requires chemotherapy. *Projection* is the placing of one's own emotions onto another. For example, a nurse who is angry about her assignment tells her nurse manager that a colleague is upset about the heavy workload. *Rationalization* is used to justify ideas or feelings that feel illogical with seemingly reasonable explanations. For example, the patient with a 60 pack/year smoking history develops lung cancer. He explains that his disease happened because he used a wood stove to heat his house. Nurses may also use defense mechanisms to preserve their self-respect, reduce feelings of guilt and anxiety, minimize distress, or maintain social acceptance by their peers.

Understanding how patients and nurses use these mechanisms to protect themselves allows for greater acceptance of the range of the human responses to stressful circumstances and more evolved approaches to communication. Carl Rogers (1961) explored the client-centered, or patient-centered, relationship and emphasized the healing powers of a successful, therapeutic relationship. He identified two essential characteristics in the helper or nurse: genuineness and unconditional positive regard or respect.

Genuineness refers to the ability to be one's own self while being a professional. Responding to a comical remark with laughter, expressing condolences to a patient suffering loss, and being humble when at a loss for answers are examples of genuineness. Self-revelations, when used appropriately and sparingly, may make the nurse appear more human and approachable so that the patient feels more comfortable revealing parts of himself or herself to the nurse. However, they must be used carefully to maintain patient-centered communication.

Unconditional positive regard or *respect* is the ability to accept patients' beliefs and attitudes despite nurses' personal feelings about them. Patients have to adapt to their health and environment in their own ways, using strategies that have worked in the past. As an example, suppose a patient with a current substance abuse problem has now tested positive for human immunodeficiency virus (HIV). While it might be challenging to care for this patient because of his ongoing risky behaviors, the nurse's job is to separate her personal reactions from the patient's situation. Interventions may include helping the patient adapt, teaching about high-risk behaviors, and encouraging health-promoting behaviors to prevent further spread of the virus.

Erik Erikson (1902–1994) described the stages of personality development as a lifelong process (Table 2-1). The eight stages of this process occur in a linear manner over time and can be influenced by social and environmental forces (Erikson, 1969). The positive resolution of each stage concludes with the acquisition of a virtue (such as hope, will, purpose, fidelity, love, and caring) and allows for normal growth and development and passage into the next stage. Society reinforces the successful achievement of the stages with ceremonies such as weddings, graduations, and retirement parties. Understanding these stages allows the nurse to understand where patients are developmentally in their lives.

As people mature, they develop more complex social skills. Life crises such as the death of a loved one or a new illness might affect the mastery of particular developmental tasks. The passage to the next stage might be more difficult or arrested, or regression to a previous stage might occur. A child who experiences the divorce of his or her parents during muscular–anal stage, for example, may

Table 2-1 Erikson's Stages of Personality Development

Stage	Critical Task to Be Accomplished	Qualities	Age
Oral–sensory	Trust versus mistrust	To receive, to give	0 to 2 years
Muscular–anal	Autonomy	To control, to let go	2 to 4 years
Locomotor–genital	Initiative versus guilt	To make, to play act	4 to 6 years
Latency	Industry versus inferiority	To make things, to put things together	6 to 12 years
Puberty	Identity versus role confusion	To be one's self	Adolescence 13 to 19 years
Young adult	Intimacy versus isolation	To share one's self with another	20 to 30 years
Adult	Generativity versus stagnation	To take care of, to create	30 to 60 years
Maturity	Integrity versus despair	To accept being, to accept not being	60 plus years

regress from being toilet trained to having accidents. As he or she adapts to the changes in his or her life, the child will regain control and move to the next stage of development. While the development of identity or self is a central life process, unexpected life circumstances such as illness are threads in the tapestry of each person's life. Erikson's theory provides a view of life as a rich, unique fabric with expected patterns or stages but also with a variety of colors.

Abraham Maslow (1970) was an American psychiatrist who developed a hierarchic categorization of human needs. In his model, the needs are stacked like a pyramid, with the most basic physiologic needs (food, water, and air) at the base taking precedence over higher needs (love and belonging). If the first level of needs (physiologic needs) is met, then the second level of needs, for physical safety and security, can be achieved. When the first two levels are met, humans need to feel love and belonging, such as to a family and/or community (love and belonging needs). People who feel they are a part of their community experience increased dignity, respect, and approval from others (self-esteem needs).

The fifth or highest level of human needs is self-actualization (Figure 2-1). To become self-actualized, people must have met their needs at all the other levels. At that point, they will be able to use their talents and personalities to the best of their abilities for the betterment of society. Self-actualized people are not perfect or free from fears and worries, but they do use themselves openly, allowing others to view their strengths and weaknesses and using themselves to improve the lives of others. The qualities of a self-actualized person are summarized here (adapted from Arnold & Boggs, 2007):

- Full acceptance of self and others
- Integrity of purpose
- Quality of genuineness
- Ability to get along well with others
- Strong sense of personal worth
- "Peak experiences"—moments of intense emotional meaning
- Ability to view life experiences as opportunities, not threats
- Strong desire to serve humanity
- Identification with fellow human beings

A variety of developmental theorists have considered the complexity of the self-concept. Travelbee (1971), in her early landmark work on humanism in nursing, described the self-concept as unique to each person. Inborn personality traits, ethnic heritage, and physiologic characteristics are different for each person and contribute to the human-to-human relationship model of nursing care. However, the development of self-concept can vary significantly, even within families. Siblings, for example, can experience the same family environment differently. Life experiences are unique for each person, both quantitatively and qualitatively. Theorists from many disciplines have explored self and self-concept, contributing to our understanding of human development across the life span. These ideas provide a foundation for exploring the nurse as a person and a healthcare professional.

Figure 2-1   Maslow's hierarchy of human needs

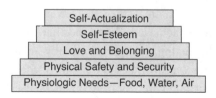

The Nurse as a Person

How do all these theories contribute to the development of a nurse? Understanding one's self as a person—the essence of self—is a lifelong goal. To paraphrase Carl Rogers (1961), people knowingly or unknowingly pursue this goal throughout life. To understand oneself allows fuller participation in life as a nurse and as a human being. To recognize and accept oneself also allows fuller acceptance of others: their strengths and weaknesses, hopes and fears, needs and desires. When the nurse fully accepts others, he or she can experience true empathy, compassion, and caring.

A person's view of the world begins with experiences within the family. Fawcett (1975) described the family as a living, open system. In family systems theory, the family is seen as a unified whole, constantly changing and reorganizing to adapt to information, energy, and matter from the surrounding environment. Every family has a unique pattern, shared values, and boundaries that separate the family from those outside the family system. Family interactions develop over time as individual family members react to one another. Ways of communicating are passed from generation to generation, and, until a member challenges the system, the communication pattern and roles persist.

No one grew up in a perfect home or with perfect parents. While small children may idolize their parents, adolescents give up these notions and begin to accept their parents as human beings. Even as adults, the memories of childhood tend to be idealized, but viewing childhood experiences through adult eyes provides insight into one's reactions to life. Communication styles also differ between family systems. Healthy families provide a safe, secure environment in which family members feel supported and valued. Members of healthy families care for one another, encourage those in need, celebrate one another's accomplishments, and openly express emotions while being considerate of the feelings of others. Rules and values are clear, and a consistent hierarchy exists. Healthy family communication allows for the expression of feelings and beliefs.

In troubled or unhealthy families, the adult members might be strictly authoritarian or unavailable to parent the children, either physically or emotionally. They may avoid anger and confrontation, or be overly controlling, openly hostile, or even physically violent. In these families, questions from children are discouraged or considered "bad" behavior. In response, children begin to repress their natural curiosity and true feelings to avoid upsetting the parents or eliciting negative responses.

Unhealthy families can produce "early helpers," children who take on adult responsibilities while repressing their own needs and feelings. Early helpers may enter "helping" professions to meet their own conscious or unconscious needs: to receive affection, to control others, or to be depended upon. Children raised in unhealthy families may have feelings of low self-esteem, shame, and victimization. While early helpers are at higher risk for substance abuse and addiction because of a need to comfort or numb uncomfortable feelings, they also have an amazing ability to cope and survive, to grow and be brave, in situations where others may not have the strength.

Developing as a Nurse

From the time a student enrolls into a nursing program, the future nurse is developing and growing. During their formal education, student nurses learn the theoretical underpinnings and facts about anatomy and physiology, pharmacology, disease and treatment, development and health. After graduation, new nurses begin to function independently and develop their own professional style. In her classic book *From Novice to Expert: Excellence and Power in Clinical Nursing Practice* (1984), Dr. Patricia Benner describes the process of how nurses acquire skills, apply nursing knowledge, and develop clinical judgment during the years of practice. While theories and evidence from research guide their practice, nurses develop expert skills by applying this knowledge to specific situations. This requires flexibility and adaptability to assess and intervene to improve individual patient outcomes—both hallmarks of excellence in nursing practice. With proper mentoring and support, new nurses can safely develop and apply nursing skills and improve the health of patients and families.

Summary

Nurses come from a variety of family backgrounds, and their previous experiences influence who they are as people and nurses. Understanding the self as a product of a family system allows for introspection and growth. Discovering oneself is a personal journey and a lifelong process that increases the ability to genuinely interact with others. Feelings of self-worth, security, and autonomy arise from previous experiences and a sense of self-awareness. Nurses, as human beings, need to take responsibility for their personal growth, acknowledge their strengths, accept their weaknesses, and incorporate strategies for self-care. Self-acceptance allows nurses to be more sensitive and compassionate. Do not be afraid to look inside to discover goals and fears, loves and needs, strengths and weaknesses—they are present in all of us, creating uniqueness in each one of us. Understanding oneself allows nurses to be effective and caring providers, combining skill, knowledge, and compassion with unique personal qualities.

Case Study Resolution

Susan was caught by surprise when Alyssa asked the question, "Are you hurt?" Susan responded, "No, I am not hurt. How are you feeling?" Susan held back her tears and finished caring for Alyssa, dressing her in her favorite rainbow pajamas. After she returned to the nurses' station, Susan sought out her instructor and asked to talk with her privately. Susan started to cry and talked about how hard it was to care for Alyssa. Susan had a niece about the same age as Alyssa who was well, but that fact still made her think about Alyssa's illness. The instructor was supportive, telling Susan that sometimes situations with patients remind the nurse of personal relationships. Separating personal from professional feelings is an important and sometimes difficult part of being a nurse. Susan had developed a good relationship with Alyssa, making her comfortable and even making her laugh about the silly pictures they had drawn together. After thought and some coaching from her instructor, Susan decided to continue caring for Alyssa that day. On Susan's return to the unit the following week, she learned that Alyssa's fever had resolved on antibiotics and she had been discharged home to her family.

EXERCISES

1. a. Complete the following statements confidentially. This exercise will help you honestly look at some aspects of yourself. It might take a week to complete this exercise, but take your time and see what you know (and don't know) about yourself.

I would describe myself as . . .
My family would describe me as . . .
My friends think I am . . .
I am proudest of . . .
I get angry when . . .

I am happy when . . .
The characteristic I most like about myself is . . .
Sometimes I get embarrassed when . . .
The thing I want most to change about myself is . . .
I get most nervous about . . .
When I am under stress, I . . .
I think that most people are . . .
The characteristic I most dislike in others is . . .
The best parts of my communication style are . . .
The parts of my communication style that I need to improve are . . .
My goals for this course are . . .
My goals for the next 5 years are . . .

b. After you complete all the statements, write a description of yourself. Who are you now? What do you like about yourself? What would you change? Which personal qualities will make you a good nurse? Which behaviors will you need to observe and change to be a more effective nurse?

2. On a piece of paper, take 5 minutes to make a timeline of the six major events in your life so far. Label each milestone according to Erickson's scheme. Then take 5 minutes to answer the following questions:
   a. According to the theorist Erik Erikson's stages of personality development, which stage are you in?
   b. Looking at Maslow's hierarchy of needs, which of your needs are met and not met?
   c. Do you know someone who is self-actualized? Describe the qualities that this person possesses.

Break into groups of three and share one answer each to one of the questions. For example, you might share your timeline or your description of a self-actualized person. Now, return to the whole group and share your responses. Which are the most common milestones on the lifelines? Do certain milestones have overlap with Erikson's stages of personality development? Which characteristics do the self-actualized people the group has described have in common? Write these qualities on the board for all to see.

Evidence-Based Article

Cowin, L. S., & Hengstberger-Sims, C. (2006). New graduate nurse self-concept and retention: a longitudinal survey. *International Journal of Nursing Studies, 43*(1), 59–70. doi: 10.1016/j.ijnurstu.2005.03.004

New nurses develop a self-concept after graduation during their first year of employment. How nurses develop this self-concept is an important predictor of retention in their first job. New nurses require support and monitoring during the first year after graduation to facilitate the growth of their new role and identify problems to improve retention.

References

Arnold, E. C., & Boggs, K. U. (2011). *Interpersonal relationships: Professional communication skills for nurses* (6th ed.). St. Louis, MO: Elsevier Saunders.

Benner, P. (1984). *From novice to expert: Excellence and power in clinical nursing practice.* Saddle River, NJ: Prentice Hall Health.

Erikson, E. (1969). *Identity and the life cycle.* New York: W. W. Norton.

Fawcett, J. (1975). The family as a living open system: An emerging conceptual framework for nursing. *International Nursing Review, 22,* 113.

Fawcett, J., & Desanto-Madeya, S. (2012) *Contemporary nursing knowledge: Analysis and evaluation of nursing models and theories.* Philadelphia, PA: F. A. Davis Company.

Freud, S. (1937). *The basic writings of Sigmund Freud.* (A.A. Brill, Trans/ed). New York: Common Library.

Maslow, A. (1970). *Motivation and personality* (2nd ed.). New York: Harper & Row.

Peplau, H. (1992). Interpersonal relations: A theoretical framework for application in practice. *Nursing Science Quarterly, 5*(1), 13–18.

Rogers, C. (1961). *On becoming a person.* Boston: Houghton Mifflin.

Sullivan, H. S. (1953). *The interpersonal theory of psychiatry.* New York: Norton.

Travelbee, J. (1971). *Interpersonal aspects of nursing.* Philadelphia, PA: F.A. Davis Company.

CHAPTER THREE

Patients as People: Standards to Guide Communication

Lisa Kennedy Sheldon

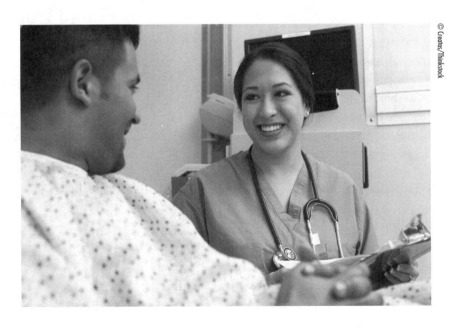

■ CASE STUDY

Mr. A. is a 67-year-old man with many physical problems. He has chronic obstructive pulmonary disease from an 80 pack/year smoking history. Plagued with arteriosclerosis, he recently suffered a stroke as well as a myocardial infarction. After his discharge from the hospital, he was transferred to a skilled nursing facility, where he was visited by the parish nurse from his local church. Despite his stroke, Mr. A. is very aware of the gravity of his health problems. The physician has told Mr. A. that his chances of returning home are slim and that his long-term prognosis is very poor. In addition, his family has told him that he cannot smoke anymore and they will no longer bring him cigarettes.

During a recent visit, the parish nurse was preparing to leave when she asked Mr. A. if there was anything she could do for him. He responded, "All I want is a cigarette. I know that I am never going to get out of this place. I have made my peace with God and I am ready to go. All I want is a cigarette. Could you bring me one?" What should the nurse do?

Introduction

The primary goal of the nurse–patient relationship is the health, well-being, and safety of the patient (American Nurses Association [ANA], 2001). When a patient and a nurse begin a relationship, a unique agreement takes place. Patients accept nurses' care with the understanding that they have their best interests in mind. Nurses and patients decide on the appropriate interventions based on an understanding of patient rights, professional standards, ethical principles, and legal statutes. Professional nurses combine these guiding factors with the patient's values and beliefs so that they can mutually determine the goals of the encounter.

Communication in nursing is guided by ethical principles, professional guidelines, and legal statutes.

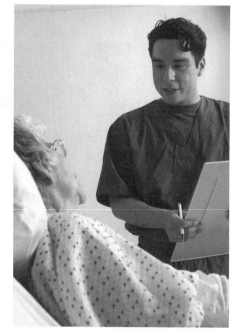
© Creatas/Thinkstock

Patient Rights

The terms "healthcare consumer," "client," and "patient" are often used preferentially in healthcare-related articles and books. A healthcare consumer is often described as one who purchases services from a healthcare provider. The more common terms, "patient" and "client," have slightly different meanings and benefit from further definition. *Merriam-Webster's Collegiate Dictionary* (1996) provides definitions for these terms:

- **Client**: One who is under the protection of another, or a person who engages the professional advice or services of another.
- **Patient**: An individual awaiting or under medical care or treatment, or one that is acted upon, derived from "one who suffers."

Because patients are in vulnerable positions that require levels of trust and vigilance from healthcare providers, the term "patient" is used in this text. For example, a patient may be medicated, unconscious, or anesthetized and cannot choose or monitor the care he or she receives while in a compromised state. Nurses and other healthcare providers make decisions collaboratively with family members in the patient's best interests. Patients trust their healthcare providers to intervene on their behalf. With a conscious patient, information must be presented in a way that facilitates patient understanding. Often, the nurse is called upon to help patients and families interpret information and assist with the decision-making process. This is an important responsibility, with moral and ethical obligations. While acknowledging that patients are also protected, the term "patient" is used in this text to symbolize the active and sometimes passive roles that patients assume while receiving health care.

The nursing profession has traditionally believed in the worth and dignity of all people seeking or requiring nursing care. The ethical principle of *self-determination* or *autonomy* guides nursing interventions and serves as the basis for informed decision making. Self-determination has its roots in the ethical tradition of *respect for persons*. Patients have the right to determine what will and will not be done to/for/with them in healthcare settings. Nurses show respect for patients by helping them remain autonomous. For example, during the decision-making process, nurses provide information that is understandable to patients while helping them weigh the benefits and side effects of treatment and presenting all options, which may include the patient's decision not to have treatment.

Advance directives are another example of patients' right to make choices about their health care. Resuscitation decisions such as a "do not resuscitate" (DNR) orders and documents for durable power of attorney are examples of *advance care directives*; such directives are established by patients prior to circumstances that could limit their ability to make these choices. Nurses, based on these ethical and legal principles, encourage patients to review their rights and make decisions about potential interventions before a health crisis occurs.

Institutional Standards

During the 1960s, a movement emerged to make the healthcare system more responsive to patients' needs. It arose in response to the public's desire to improve the quality of health care and hold healthcare institutions and providers more accountable for the outcomes of care. Today patients are assuming more responsibility for their own health and adopting preventive health behaviors, such as adequate exercise and healthy eating (primary prevention). Healthcare providers such as nurses share in this responsibility when they educate both patients and the community about primary prevention and early detection (e.g., via screening such as mammography and colonoscopy). The provider and the patient share in the responsibility for determining the best care for each patient.

In response to this movement, the American Hospital Association published "A Patient's Bill of Rights" in 1973 (revised in 1992). Its purpose continues to be to promote the rights of patients. Today hospitals have adopted this document as part of entrance into a healthcare setting, providing each patient with a printed copy.

The Patient's Bill of Rights includes the following important components:

- The right to considerate and respectful care
- The right to privacy, including confidentiality of all records of the patient's care
- The right to make decisions about the patient's care, including the right to refuse care or treatment
- The right to review all medical records and have them explained
- The right to refuse to participate in research studies

- The right to make statements about the patient's care, including a living will and advance care directives
- The right to be informed of resources in the hospital to resolve disputes or grievances

While many of these rights appear to be common sense, they were never formally adopted or documented until the 1970s. Many insurance companies and health maintenance organizations also offer bills of rights to their patients. The Health Insurance Portability and Accountability Act of 1996 (HIPAA Privacy Rule) set national standards regarding the privacy of certain health information to protect people who seek care and healing in the healthcare system. The compliance of a healthcare provider or facility with HIPAA regulations is often defined in handouts that are provided to all patients. In both the Patient's Bill of Rights and HIPAA documents, the same themes emerge about patient care and communication that have roots in ethical traditions—namely, respect, autonomy, and privacy.

Professional Standards

Nurses, as healthcare professionals, are required to adhere to the scope of their knowledge and practice. The American Nurses Association wrote the Code of Ethics for Nurses to define the nursing role (ANA, 1973, 1991, 2001, 2004). The Code of Ethics highlights the roles filled by nurses, including their primary commitment to the patient and advocacy for the health, safety and rights of all patients. The ANA's Social Policy Statement (2010) also defines nursing's value to society and the scope and standards of practice. These important guidelines not only establish the scope of nursing practice and the level of performance of nursing services, but also serve as the standards by which nurses are held accountable by the public and the judicial system. Additionally, they are the basis for state Nurse Practice Acts, the legal documents approved by each state's legislature that describe the scope of nursing practice, including nurses' rights, responsibilities, and licensure requirements. *Scope of practice* refers to legal and ethical parameters of nursing practice, including direct care (such as administration of medications), coordination of care with other disciplines, and delegation of care to other personnel (such as nursing assistants). A board of nursing in each state in the United States oversees nursing practice. Specialty practice guidelines provide additional instruction for specific clinical areas, such as pediatrics or geriatrics.

Legal Standards

Laws define the boundaries and expectations of the nursing profession. Legal statutes serve to protect the public and set the standards for professional nursing care. The legal standard known as "a reasonable standard of care" is based in tort law; it is defined as care that a reasonably prudent nurse would provide in a similar situation. The reasonable standard of care is used as a benchmark in courts of law to judge criminal negligence. It holds a nurse accountable for his or her actions or failure to act. Criminal negligence by a nurse includes failing to protect a patient from harm, performing a nursing action that a reasonably prudent nurse would not perform, or failing to perform an action that a reasonably prudent nurse would perform. For example, if a nurse hears a patient talking about methods to kill himself and does nothing to protect the patient from harming himself, then this failure to act is criminally negligent behavior. Other examples of unprofessional conduct include breaching patient confidentiality, performing actions without sufficient preparation, failing to report or document changes in a patient's status, verbally or physically abusing a patient, and falsifying records.

Confidentiality

Patient confidentiality is an important issue from a professional, legal, and institutional point of view. Confidentiality stems from the ethical tradition of the right to privacy. Breaching a patient's confidential communication is a breach of trust and violates standards established by institutions and the government. Standards from the Office of Civil Rights/Health Insurance Portability and Accountability Act of 1996 (OCR/HIPAA) define the protection of patients' individually identifiable data arising from encounters with healthcare services. Specifically, only information that is pertinent to the patient's treatment may be shared with other healthcare providers. Moreover, only those providers who have a "need to know" may be given specific information. For example, if a worker sustained a back injury on the job, then only health information related to the injury would be given to the insurer in relation to a worker's compensation claim, not the entire medical record.

Legally, communication between a nurse and a patient is considered to be privileged communication, and the law forbids the nurse from disclosing this information, with one exception. If this communication includes evidence that could harm innocent people, including the patient, then, legally and morally, this information must be shared with the appropriate authorities. Included in this exception are instances of child abuse, gunshot wounds, and communicable diseases.

Communication and Malpractice

Within the realm of legal issues pertaining to nursing practice lies the issue of malpractice. While it might be difficult to understand why a text that focuses on talking with patients would address this issue, good communication may be one of the best ways to prevent clinical problems from being cited as reasons for claims of malpractice (Levinson et al., 1997). Even while working within the scope of nursing practice and maintaining excellent clinical skills, nurses may encounter patients who are angry or dissatisfied with their care. Nurses may be named in lawsuits, despite providing the best nursing care. Conversely, patients who feel that they were treated with respect and compassion sue healthcare providers less frequently (Levinson et al., 1997). Also, patients who feel that their providers really listen to them are usually satisfied patients. Good "bedside manner" is not just a secondary part of being a nurse; it is essential to good nursing practice, improves the accuracy of assessments, creates effective interventions, prevents complications, and produces more satisfied patients. Thus the same basic concepts of good communication—respect, empathy, and genuineness—may also prevent malpractice claims (Box 3-1).

Box 3-1   Communication Skills to Prevent Malpractice Claims

- Be respectful and genuine.
- Listen to what patients say and don't say, striving to understand their experiences.
- Be available and accessible.
- Avoid rote phrases that might demean what the patient is saying.
- Be clear about the reasoning used to reach decisions regarding the patient's care.
- Involve the patient in decision making and the informed consent process.
- Carry through with commitments to patients and do not make promises that cannot be kept.
- Be honest about what is known and what requires further research or consultation.

Values

Moral reasoning and decision making require the ability to identify values—specifically, the nurse's values and the patient's values. As discussed in the chapter titled *The Nurse as a Person: Theories of Self and Nursing*, the nurse brings a set of values to the professional role. Some values come from one's cultural and ethnic background. (See the *Cross-Cultural Communication* chapter for more on cultural diversity.) Others are based on personal experiences, beliefs, and attitudes. Throughout life, values are acquired from family, friends, religious groups, and the community. It is important that the nurse delivers care in a manner that respects the patient's values and needs. It is also vital that the nurse identifies and respects the patient's values even if these values differ from his or her own.

Values are a person's beliefs about the truth, beauty, and worth of any thought, object, or behavior. They give direction and meaning to life and guide the decision-making process. Values also determine behavior by guiding the responses to experiences and choices in life. Nurses need to be aware and conscious of the values that influence patients' behaviors and perceptions, and respect patients' abilities to make choices about their own health care. Nurses need to focus on patients' needs based on their values, while recognizing that these needs and values may be different from the nurse's own values. Nurses who develop awareness of their own values are better able to provide respectful, patient-centered care.

Code of Ethics for Nurses

To establish a profession, an ethical code must be formulated. The nursing profession, through the ANA, developed the Code of Ethics for Nurses with Interpretive Statements (1976, 1985, 2001) to delineate the expectations of ethical nursing practice and acknowledge the responsibility entrusted in the nursing profession by the public. The Code of Ethics for Nurses makes the following assertions:

- The nurse, in all professional relationships, practices with compassion and respect for the inherent dignity, worth, and uniqueness of every individual, unrestricted by considerations of social or economic status, personal attributes, or the nature of health problems.
- The nurse's primary commitment is to the patient, whether an individual, family, group, or community.
- The nurse promotes, advocates for, and strives to protect the health, safety, and rights of the patient.

- The nurse is responsible and accountable for individual nursing practice and determines the appropriate delegation of tasks consistent with the nurse's obligation to provide optimum patient care.
- The nurse owes the same duties to self as to others, including the responsibility to preserve integrity and safety, to maintain competence, and to continue personal and professional growth.
- The nurse participates in establishing, maintaining, and improving healthcare environments and conditions of employment conducive to the provision of quality health care and consistent with the values of the profession through individual and collective action.
- The nurse participates in the advancement of the profession through contributions to practice, education, administration, and knowledge development.
- The nurse collaborates with other health professionals and the public in promoting community, national, and international efforts to meet health needs.
- The profession of nursing as represented by associations and their members is responsible for articulating nursing values, for maintaining the integrity of the profession and its practice, and for shaping public policy.[*]

The Code of Ethics for Nurses is a published and public document of nursing practice that should drive and guide all nursing care. The code also outlines the public's expectations of the services provided by a professional nurse.

Ethical Reasoning and Decision Making

Ethical reasoning serves to guide decision making in the nurse–patient relationship and the implementation of the decision in practice. There are often multiple ways to view an ethical dilemma and often no one right decision. Three decision-making models may be used to view a situation:

1. Utilitarian or goal-based model: The "rightness" of an action is based on the consequences and contribution to the overall goodness of an action.
2. Deontological or duty-based model: The "rightness" of an action is based on other factors besides goodness, including respect for the person, the rights of the individual, and best interests of the patient.
3. Human rights–based model: The "rightness" of an action is based on the rights of the patient. (Arnold & Boggs, 2007, pp. 47–48)

Nurses may use all three models at different times depending on the patient and the situation. Ethical dilemmas arise when conflicts develop, such as between professional and personal values, professional values and laws, and the nurse's values and the patient's values, or between professions. Nurses require support during ethical decisions so they can advocate for patients and not conform to the decisions of others (Goethals, Gastmans, & de Casterlé, 2010).

Resolution of ethical dilemmas is often guided by three ethical principles: autonomy, beneficence, and justice. *Autonomy* is the patient's right to self-determination. *Beneficence* denotes that an action must result in the greatest good for the patient. Conversely, nonmaleficence refers to actions that "do no harm" to the patient and is the basis of the Hippocratic Oath. *Justice* refers to actions and decisions being fair and/or impartial. While it is often used as a legal term, justice may also refer to the equitable distribution of resources, the determination of social worth of patients, and the veracity or truthfulness that is inherent in the nurse–patient relationship. Veracity and trust imply that the nurse cannot lie to the patient, but questions remain about whether a nurse may withhold information that might cause a patient distress.

Helping patients to arrive at decisions about their care is a fundamental component of the nurse's role. This decision making is guided by the patient's values and beliefs as the nurse helps the patient to identify these values as well as potential conflicts and the desired goals (Box 3-2). The focus of decision making needs to be the patient's goals. It is important that nurses separate their own values and

---

Box 3-2 Steps in Ethical Decision Making

- Gather background information: Collect known information about the patient and the context of the situation.
- Identify ethical components: Recognize the underlying issues and who will be affected by the decision.
- Clarify roles: Know the rights and obligations of all involved parties.
- Explore options: Investigate alternatives, potential negative effects, goals, and desired outcomes.
- Apply ethical principles: Consider ethical theories and scientific facts.
- Resolve the dilemma: Understand the effects of the decision, implement the action, and determine how the outcomes will be evaluated.

goals from those of their patients to facilitate communication and support the patient. Frequently there may be more than one right decision, requiring more discussion, time, and patience to resolve the issue, but the focus always remains on the patient's right to choose. Often, difficult decisions also bring emotional reactions, making the decision-making process more complex. Nurses work to support patients' rights by interpreting information, providing support and clarification, and helping patients to prioritize and make informed choices.

Summary

People enter a healthcare setting with certain rights and individual values. Institutions, professions, and government authorities protect the rights of the person receiving health care as a patient by creating standards, guidelines, codes of ethics, and laws. In the profession of nursing, guidelines for practice are published by state and national nursing organizations and serve to guide professionals and provide public declaration of the standards of a profession. The goal of all guidelines, ethical principles, and legal statutes is to protect the patient. Incorporating professional guidelines with the ethical principles and the patient's values allows for nursing care that is unique, respectful, and effective for each patient.

Case Study Resolution

The parish nurse thought about how to respond to Mr. A. She considered her beliefs about smoking and health, her long-term relationship with Mr. A., and his prognosis. His health condition was very poor, and his future life was limited by his chronic obstructive pulmonary disease (COPD), renal failure, and recent stroke and heart attack. It would bring him pleasure to have a cigarette and probably would not change his prognosis. Focusing on compassionate care and respect for this patient as a person, the parish nurse decided to bring Mr. A. a pack of cigarettes. He was very grateful and asked the nurse to roll his wheelchair outside so he could smoke. In the spring air, they talked about his life and what had made him happy over the years: his son, his garden, and his friends in a fraternal order. When the parish nurse left the nursing home that spring afternoon, she felt that she had made the right decision by bringing the cigarettes for Mr. A.

Mr. A. died 4 weeks later as the result of a urinary tract infection and renal failure.

EXERCISES

VALUE PRIORITY EXERCISE

This exercise is aimed at increasing self-awareness and clarifying values. Complete this exercise privately.

Read through the following list of values and rate their level of importance to you:

1. Very important
2. Important
3. Not important

After completion, pick out the five highest-rated values and the five values with the lowest scores. Remember, there is no right or wrong answer. Try to be honest with yourself.

VALUES

- Achievement (accomplishment)
- Aesthetics (appreciation of beauty in art and nature)
- Altruism (service to others, interest in the well-being of others)
- Autonomy (personal freedom, self-determination)
- Creativity (developing new ideas)
- Emotional well-being (peace of mind, inner security)
- Health (physical and mental well-being)
- Honesty (being truthful and genuine)
- Justice (treating others fairly)
- Knowledge (pursuit of information, truth, principles)
- Love (caring, unselfish devotion)
- Loyalty (allegiance to a person or group)
- Morality (honor, integrity, keeping ethical standards)
- Physical appearance (concern for one's appearance, being well-groomed)
- Pleasure (fun, joy, gratification, enjoying life)
- Power (control, authority, influence over others)
- Recognition (being important, well-liked)
- Spirituality (having a religious belief)
- Wealth (having possessions or enough money)
- Wisdom (mature understanding, insight, good judgment)

Five Most Important Values

1.

2.

3.

4.

5.

Five Least Important Values

1.

2.

3.

4.

5.

Evidence-Based Article

Solum, E. M., Maluwa, V. M., & Severinsson, E. (2012). Ethical problems in practice as experienced by Malawian student nurses. *Nursing Ethics, 19*(1), 128–138. doi: 10.1177/0969733011412106

Student nurses often see ethical challenges in clinical practice. This study explored Malawian students' perceptions of ethical problems during clinical experiences. Ten nursing students were interviewed. In this study, the researchers found three main themes emerged: (1) conflict between patient rights and the guardians' presence in the hospital; (2) conflict between violation of professional values and patient rights caused by unethical behavior; and (3) conflict between moral awareness and the ideal course of action. The authors also found that students had difficulty ensuring patient rights and acting in accordance with Western norms and values. These values may not be appropriate in the Malawian culture. The researchers suggest that students would benefit from role models who demonstrate professional attitudes toward patients' rights and values. There is also a need to teach students ethical reflection during clinical practice.

References

American Nurses Association. (2001). Code of ethics for nurses with interpretive statements. Retrieved from http://www.nursingworld.org/MainMenuCategories/EthicsStandards/ CodeofEthicsforNurses/Code-of-Ethics.pdf

American Nurses Association. (2010). Nursing's social policy statement. Foundation of nursing package. Retrieved from http://www.nursesbooks.org/Main-Menu/Foundation/Nursings-Social-Policy-Statement.aspx

Arnold, E., & Boggs, K. U. (2007). Clinical judgment: Applying critical thinking and ethical decision making. In *Interpersonal relationships: Professional communication skills for nurses* (5th ed.). Philadelphia: W. B. Saunders.

Goethals, S., Gastmans, C., & de Casterlé, B. D. (2010). Nurses' ethical reasoning and behaviour: A literature review. *International Journal of Nursing Studies, 47*(5), 635–650. doi: 10.1016/j.ijnurstu.2009.12.010

Levinson, W., Roter, D., Mulloly, J. P., et al. (1997). Physician-patient communication: The relationship with malpractice claims among primary care physicians and surgeons. *Journal of the American Medical Association, 277*, 553–559.

Merriam-Webster's Collegiate Dictionary (1996). (10th ed.). Springfield, MA: Merriam-Webster, Inc.

Stuart, G. W., & Sundeen, S. J. (1991). *Principles and practice of psychiatric nursing* (4th ed.). St. Louis, MO: Mosby Elsevier.

CHAPTER FOUR

Cross-Cultural Communication

Judith Healey Walsh

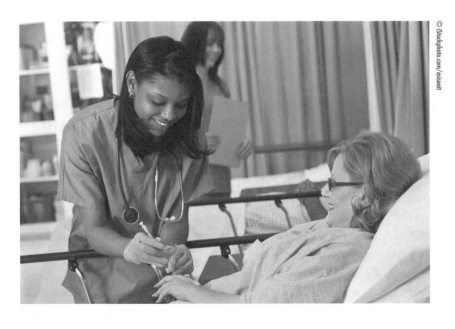

■ CASE STUDY

Mrs. R. is a 35-year-old, Spanish-speaking, Colombian female who presented at the emergency room (ER) with her 12-year-old son, who appeared to be bilingual. Enlisting the son to interpret, the nurse determined that the patient had experienced nausea and vomiting this morning and for the past few days. She also seemed to have some stomach cramping. The ER had been treating many patients with symptoms of a stomach virus over the past few days, and the nurse and physician determined that Mrs. R. was suffering from the same virus. The nurse did note that Mrs. R. was holding her abdomen, moaning, and seemed to be in more pain than other patients, but she knew that Latino patients are very emotive and demonstrative in response to pain, so the nurse minimized the importance of this reaction and did not explore any further. The nurse felt frustrated with the patient's inability to communicate in English and focused on the son, interacting only minimally with the patient. The nurse gave the son the discharge instructions for dealing with a stomach virus, and the woman was discharged, although she seemed somewhat confused and upset.

The next day the same nurse saw that Mrs. R. had returned accompanied by her husband. The woman was hemorrhaging and in distress.

What went wrong in this cross-cultural clinical encounter? What could have been done differently?

Introduction

During the past decade, the United States has become increasingly more racially, ethnically, and culturally diverse. In 2010, African American, Hispanic, Asian, and Native populations accounted for 35% of the nation's 308.7 million people, and these minority populations were increasing at more rapid rates than non-Hispanic Whites (U.S. Census Bureau, 2010). Yet compared to the overall U.S. population, registered nurses—who constitute the United States' largest population of healthcare professionals—are overwhelmingly White. Findings from the 2008 National Sample Survey of Registered Nurses estimated the RN workforce to be 83.2% White and 16.8% African American, Hispanic, Asian, and Native American (Health Resources and Services Administration, 2008). The demographic changes in the U.S. population have led to an increasing number of cross-cultural clinical encounters in nursing practice. Nurses in the United States are providing care for a greater proportion of patients whose cultural perspectives, experiences, attitudes, beliefs, and behaviors may be different from theirs (Calvillo et al., 2009).

As cross-cultural clinical encounters in health care have increased, issues of cultural misunderstandings, bias, prejudice, and stereotyping about race or culture have become more prevalent (Baldwin, 2003; Betancourt, Green, Carrillo, & Ananeh-Firempong, 2003). When healthcare providers, such as nurses, respond from an ethnocentric perspective, accept stereotypes, or harbor feelings of bias or prejudice toward patients based on their membership in a specific racial or ethnic group, that point of view frequently negatively influences the provider's communication with and care provided to that patient (Baldwin, 2003; Betancourt et al., 2003). The impact of bias, prejudice, and stereotyping on quality of care has been identified as a factor that contributes to persistent health disparities—that is, differences in the type of health care received and health outcomes achieved among diverse groups of people (Baldwin, 2003; Smedley, Stith, & Nelson, 2002). Even well-meaning providers who are not overtly biased may demonstrate unconscious negative cultural attitudes and stereotypes (Smedley et al., 2002).

In response to pressing concerns about health disparities and cultural misunderstandings, national educational, professional, and regulatory associations (American Association of Colleges of Nursing [AACN], 2008; Douglas et al., 2011; The Joint Commission, 2010; Smedley et al., 2002) have identified the development of cultural competence as an essential component in nursing education and practice to improve cross-cultural clinical encounters and address health disparities. The American Academy of Nursing's Expert Panel on Global Health and Nursing and Cultural Competence identified 12 Standards of Practice for Culturally Competent Nursing Care. Two of the standards are particularly relevant to cultural communication. Standard 4 relates to the development of cultural competence and states, "Nurses shall use cross-cultural knowledge and culturally sensitive skills in implementing culturally congruent care," while Standard 12 states, "Nurses shall use culturally competent verbal and nonverbal communication skills to identify client's values, beliefs, practices, perceptions, and unique healthcare needs" (Douglas et al., 2011). Increasing diversity has also prompted healthcare regulators to institute requirements related to the provision of culturally competent care.

To effectively implement these requirements, healthcare providers must accommodate their patients' cultural, religious, and personal values, beliefs, and preferences in care, treatment, and services rendered (The Joint Commission, 2010).

Patients are people arising from a variety of cultural, social, and ethnic backgrounds.

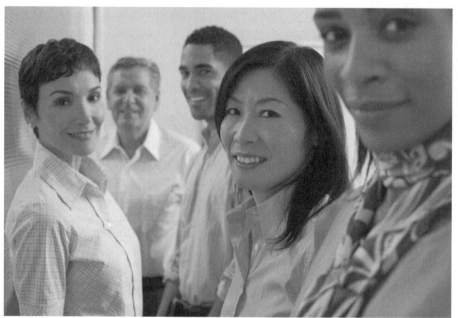

© Jupiterimages/Comstock/Thinkstock

This chapter focuses on three areas, which will contribute to your understanding of the influence that culture has on healthcare communication and the challenges inherent in cross-cultural communication: (1) a conceptual grounding of culture and cultural competence as they relate to health care; (2) barriers to effective cross-cultural communication; and (3) strategies to improve cross-cultural clinical encounters.

Culture, Cultural Competence, and Health Care

Although multiple definitions of *culture* exist, this term is commonly understood to mean the shared beliefs, values, ideas, language, communication, norms, practices, and behaviors of a group of people. An individual's values, beliefs, and practices related to health and illness are influenced by that person's culture. Despite similarities, fundamental differences among people arise from ethnicity and culture, as well as from family background and individual experience. Diverse belief systems exist related to perceptions of health and illness, their causes, and acceptable treatments. Cultural differences, in turn, affect the health beliefs, behaviors, and communication styles of both patients and providers, such as nurses. They also influence the expectations that patients and providers have for each other. These patient–provider issues substantiate the need for educational, practice, and organizational standards, competencies, policies, and practices, which support the delivery of culturally and linguistically congruent health care. The Joint Commission (2010)—the agency that accredits hospitals and other healthcare agencies—provides the following definition of cultural competence:

> Cultural competence is the ability of health care providers and health care organizations to understand and respond effectively to the cultural and language needs brought by the patient to the health care encounter. Cultural competence requires organizations and their personnel to do the following: (1) value diversity; (2) assess themselves; (3) manage the dynamics of difference; (4) acquire and institutionalize cultural knowledge; and (5) adapt to diversity and the cultural contexts of individuals and communities served. (p. 1)

Nursing education and practice have acknowledged that acquisition of knowledge, skills, and attitudes is required for the development of cultural competence. Campinha-Bacote (2002), a nurse theorist, developed a cultural competence model, known as the process of cultural competence in the delivery of healthcare services, which comprises five interrelated constructs: (1) cultural awareness, (2) cultural knowledge, (3) cultural skill, (4) cultural encounters, and (5) cultural desire. This model serves as a useful guide to the ongoing development of cultural competence, effective cross-cultural communication, and ultimately culturally congruent care.

Cultural awareness involves self-examination and in-depth exploration of one's own cultural and professional background. The reflective process should begin with the novice student nurse and continue through the professional development of the nurse. It leads to the recognition of the nurse's biases, prejudices, and assumptions about individuals who are perceived as culturally different from the nurse. Developing cultural knowledge involves obtaining an educational foundation pertaining to worldviews, varied definitions of health and illness, and differences in treatment preferences and treatment efficacy among different racial and ethnic groups. The ability to perform an effective culturally based assessment and physical examination, along with respectful cross-cultural communication, constitutes cultural skill. Cultural encounters provide opportunities for healthcare providers to engage in cross-cultural interactions, which in turn help providers to modify or refine their existing beliefs about a cultural group, with the intention of preventing possible stereotyping. Such encounters can help the provider realize the extent of intraethnic variation—that is, variation within a cultural group as opposed to variation across cultural groups. Finally, Campinha-Bacote (2002) describes cultural desire as "the motivation to *want* to rather than *have* to engage in cultural encounters" (p. 182). She notes that "cultural desire includes genuine passion to be open and flexible with others, to accept differences and build on similarities, and to be willing to learn from others as cultural informants" (p. 183).

Barriers to Effective Cross-Cultural Communication

Effective communication between patients and healthcare providers, such as nurses, is a significant factor with regard to patient safety, patient satisfaction, and the quality of nursing care (Ardoin & Wilson, 2010; Jirwe, Gerrish, & Emami, 2010). Communication is a complex process comprising much more than just a linguistic component. It requires the interpretation of speech, tone, facial expressions, gestures, and assumptions shared between the provider and the patient about the context and purpose of the exchange. Culture influences all aspects of communication, and when the clinical encounter crosses cultures, the potential for misunderstandings, reduced patient satisfaction, poorer health outcomes, and possible adverse events increases (Cioffi, 2003; Jirwe et al., 2010). This section outlines the primary barriers to satisfactory cross-cultural communication in clinical encounters.

Lack of Cultural Awareness and Knowledge

First, nurses may lack awareness or understanding of their own cultural values, beliefs, and behaviors and the potential influence they exert in their interactions with patients. Second, nurses may lack knowledge and understanding of how patients' cultures shape their understanding of what constitutes health and illness and how they respond to each of these states. Third, lack of awareness and understanding of how culture shapes communication modes and influences the nurse–patient encounter can lead to misunderstandings, mistrust, and poor patient outcomes. Culture is one aspect that dictates what is considered normal behavior when an individual is ill, yet if nurses are unaware of cultural differences they may expect all patients to react in a similar manner.

Ethnocentrism

Ethnocentrism—a universal tendency—occurs when an individual believes that her or his cultural values, beliefs, and practices are the best and superior to those of individuals from another culture. This tendency can lead nurses to impose their cultural preferences onto the care provided for the patient, while ignoring and denigrating the patient's cultural values, beliefs, practices, and preferences.

Bias and Prejudice

Beyond ethnocentric tendencies, nurses may harbor either overt or unconscious biases about people from other racial or cultural groups that influence their interactions and nursing care. Based on previous or ongoing experiences with discrimination (action based on prejudice), patients may have developed a distrust of healthcare providers or institutions. Trust is essential in patient–provider relationships; without trust, open, honest, and effective communication is significantly hindered.

Nurses educated in the United States frequently demonstrate a strong bias toward the Western, biomedical healthcare system in which they were educated. This system emphasizes a biological basis for disease and a rational approach to treatment. When nurses believe that the biomedical system is the best—and possibly the only—approach to patient care, they may view other health belief systems, which incorporate herbal medicines, traditional and folk healers, and culturally based illness etiologies, as substandard and lacking merit and, therefore, communicate a condescending, rigid, and controlling attitude. This attitude will alienate patients who feel that their beliefs and preferences have been ignored and disrespected. Communication will break down, with patients no longer sharing information regarding their health beliefs and practices, potentially ignoring the nurse's advice and treatment plan, and perhaps not returning for follow-up or subsequent care.

Stereotyping

Typically nursing students learn about other cultures through a categorical approach, which focuses on the presentation of relevant values, attitudes, health beliefs, and behaviors associated with specific cultures. For example, lists of health beliefs and practices, along with do's and don'ts specific to the health care of various cultural groups, such as Vietnamese or Mexicans, are often provided to students.

However, this approach tends to ignore the significant variations that occur within cultural groups (Betancourt et al., 2003) and has been shown to lead to stereotyping (Campinha-Bacote, 2002). When facing increasing cultural diversity among patient populations, it might seem simpler and more efficient to categorize patients according to their primary cultural affiliation—but this strategy ignores intra-ethnic variation as well as the multiple intersecting background factors, including race, ethnicity, social class, age, and gender, that shape any particular individual's identity. Communication and nursing care that are based on unexamined stereotypes will most likely lead to misunderstandings and unsatisfactory outcomes.

Lack of Understanding of Key Cultural Characteristics

Key cultural characteristics—such as whether a culture emphasizes individualistic or collectivistic values or is predominantly high or low context—strongly influence communication styles, accounting for significant variations among different groups (Hall, 1976). A lack of understanding of these potential differences can block effective communication between the nurse and patient.

In general, high-context cultures (e.g., Asian, African, and Latin American) tend to be collectivist, emphasizing group needs and consensus over individual desires and decisions. There is a strong emphasis on interpersonal relationships, with the establishment of trust being foundational to effective communication. Communication may be indirect, with words not being as important as context, which may include the speaker's tone of voice, facial expression, gestures, posture, and status. Intuition and contemplation may be valued more than reason and logic. Saving face and maintaining harmony are important components within communication, confrontation may be avoided, and authority is respected.

In contrast, low-context cultures (e.g., North American and Western European) tend to value the individual and his or her autonomy. These cultures are goal and action oriented, with an emphasis on assertiveness, logic, and rationality. Communication is direct; words are most important (with context contributing much less to the communication) and are expected to be clear, precise, and taken literally. There is a desire to get right to the task or action, with less need to personally interact.

Differences in these communication styles can prove highly problematic within clinical encounters. Nurses socialized in low-context cultures may be perceived by a patient from a high-context culture as curt, disinterested, unfeeling, and even rude if the nurse moves too quickly to intrusive questions or tasks without spending time to establish rapport, or if the nurse's facial expression, posture, or tone reveals unintentional signs of frustration or condescension. The nurse may also misinterpret the patient's minimal verbal responses and unwillingness to make independent decisions as being intentionally vague, uncooperative, and avoidant.

Language Barriers

When patients do not speak the nurse's language or have limited English proficiency, communication can be particularly challenging. Studies have revealed that nurses and patients find these communication situations frustrating, and both parties report the provision of care to be less satisfying (Cioffi, 2003). In such situations, nurses sometimes use untrained interpreters such as family members, friends, and bilingual support staff to facilitate communication. Yet for interpretation to be successful, the interpreter needs to have a high degree of proficiency in both languages and possess special interactive skills. Studies have found the following problems when family members and friends are used as interpreters: (1) lack of familiarity with medical terminology in either language, (2) deletion of

During nurse–patient interactions, the patient is the "cultural informant."

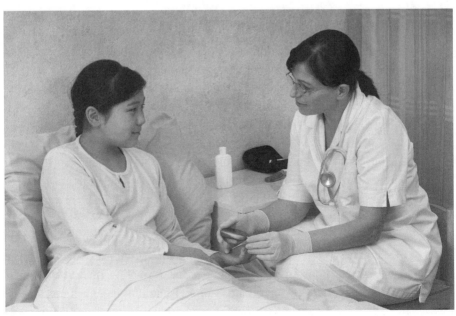

© iStockphoto/Thinkstock

important information because they cannot keep up, (3) modification of meaning because they cannot make a literal translation, (4) omission of pertinent sexual or sensitive information by the patient or family interpreter due to embarrassment, and (5) breach in confidentiality; these problems may lead to serious miscommunication and medical errors (Flores et al., 2003; Rivadeneyra, Elderkin-Thompson, Silver, & Waitzkin, 2000).

Strategies to Improve Cross-Cultural Clinical Encounters

It is evident that cross-cultural clinical encounters pose communication challenges for both nurses and patients. Communication difficulties can prevent the development of the rapport and trust between nurses and patients that is necessary for effective therapeutic alliances and patient-centered care. Therefore, nurses need to identify ways in which they can gain better understanding of cultural implications in nursing care and improved skill in cross-cultural communication. This section provides insights into the knowledge, skills, and attitudes that can enhance cross-cultural communication and care.

Use a Cultural Humility Approach

Tervalon and Murray-Garcia (1998) suggest that healthcare providers' use of a cultural humility approach can improve cross-cultural communication and care. First, this approach requires that the providers commit to lifelong self-evaluation and critique of their cultural values, beliefs, biases, conceptions, and preferences. This approach views the provider as continually working toward "becoming" culturally competent, which represents a lifelong journey. The ongoing reflection and critique assist providers, such as nurses, in acknowledging their biases, the potential impact those biases could have on the care that they provide, and the need to avoid cultural imposition on the patients they serve. Second, cultural humility seeks to avoid stereotyping, with the provider instead approaching the individual patient as the knowledge bearer and teacher of her or his cultural values, beliefs, practices, and preferences. Third, this strategy involves a conscious attempt on the part of the nurse to address the power imbalance that typically occurs within the nurse–patient relationship and encourages the formation of a true partnership, which fosters patient-centered care. Cultural humility demonstrates sincere respect for the patient, values each person's individual cultural perspective and preferences, and seeks to establish a collaborative and ethnosensitive rather than hierarchical and ethnocentric relationship with the patient.

Use an Inquiry Process

To approach the patient as the teacher of his or her cultural perspective and preferences, the nurse needs to engage in an inquiry process in a thoughtful, respectful, and considerate manner. Several areas of culture may have an impact on health, yet these may be overlooked in clinical encounters. The cultural norms and values that define these areas can vary significantly and if not explored can lead to misunderstandings and poor communication.

- Family perspective and involvement: Cultural norms determine how family decision-making processes are structured. The nurse should ask the patient who, if anyone, must be involved in communication and decision making other than the patient.
- Male–female roles and sexual behavior: These roles and norms for sexual behavior can vary by culture. The nurse should be alert for differences in rights and responsibilities, and any gender role restrictions, that may affect communication with healthcare professionals. The nurse should be sensitive to modesty issues and ask if there is a preference for same-gender care providers.
- Dietary beliefs and customs: Culture has a strong influence on dietary beliefs, customs, and practices as they relate to maintaining health and treating illness. Nurses need to ask patients about their dietary preferences and restrictions and respectfully integrate them into their care.
- Pain expression and management: Pain can have different meanings and be expressed differently among individuals and across cultures. Nurses need to evaluate their assumptions in relation to stereotypes about pain expression and tolerance and become open and skilled in accepting and responding to wide variation in pain expression. The nurse needs to establish a trusting environment, whereby the patient is comfortable in expressing her or his pain both verbally and nonverbally and the nurse is skillful in interpreting this expression.
- End-of-life care and decision making: Strong cultural norms shape expectations and practices around death and dying. The nurse needs to inquire about disclosure of terminal status, who is involved in decision making, who needs to be involved in providing care, and which cultural or religious rites need to be incorporated in care.

LEARN About the Patient's Perspective on Health and Illness

Kleinman, Eisenberg, and Good (1978) emphasized the importance of eliciting patients' perceptions of their own health problems as a method of gaining cultural understanding and improving cross-cultural communication. Kleinman and associates (1978, p. 256) identified the following series of questions and described them as the explanatory model of illness:

- What do you think caused your illness?
- Why do you think it started when it did?
- What do you think your sickness does to you? How does it work?
- How severe is your sickness? Will it have a short or a long course?
- Which kind of treatment do you think you should receive?
- What are the most important results you hope to receive from this treatment?
- What are the chief problems your sickness has caused for you?
- What do you fear most about your sickness?

The following is an adapted version of the LEARN mnemonic developed by Berlin and Fowkes (1983) to guide respectful, patient-centered cross-cultural communication.

L: Listen to what patients say with empathy and understanding. Listen to the patient's perception of the problem without imposing your own values and beliefs, which may conflict with those of the patient. Active listening involves attending to both verbal and nonverbal communication. Nurses must observe and become sensitive to culturally specific paralanguage variations such as voice volume, tone, intonation, eye contact, and willingness to share thoughts and feelings.

E: Explain your perceptions of the problem and express your understanding that the perception of illness and disease, its causes, and treatments vary by culture.

A: Acknowledge and discuss the differences and similarities in the perspectives and communication styles. Be careful not to devalue the patient's perspective and privilege your own perspective and preferences. Adapt your communication style to the patient's cultural context.

R: Recommend nursing care and treatments that respect individual patient preferences and integrate aspects of cultural health beliefs (e.g., herbal medicine, traditional healers, dietary customs, and cultural rituals).

N: Negotiate agreement as authentic partners (not as superior authority figure) in developing, implementing, and evaluating the plan of care.

Use Trained Interpreters

When patients do not speak English or have limited English proficiency, the use of professionally trained interpreters is considered the best practice and has been found to improve the safety and quality of care provided (Jacobs et al., 2001). Nurses should be aware of the federal, state, and accreditation regulations and standards that exist regarding provision of healthcare communication in the preferred language of the patient. Nurses should also gain skill in working with an interpreter. Key guidelines to follow when using an interpreter are listed here:

- Insist that the interpreter repeat everything that you and the patient say, emphasizing accuracy, completeness, and impartiality.
- Look at the patient, not the interpreter (have interpreter stand behind and slightly to one side of the patient).
- Express one concept at a time, pace your speech, enunciate clearly, and avoid using medical jargon and American slang.
- Occasionally ask the interpreter to tell you what he or she just said when explaining a point to a patient. This feedback will provide the opportunity to assess the quality of the translation and to identify any mistakes.
- Encourage the interpreter to ask questions when he or she is uncertain.

Summary

The population of the United States continues to become more culturally diverse. Culture exerts a strong influence on an individual's values, beliefs, practices, preferences, and behaviors related to health and illness. It is crucial to recognize that both patients and providers bring cultural perspectives to the clinical encounter, which can lead to cross-cultural challenges. Therefore, nurses need to be aware of their own cultural influences, biases, and stereotypes and commit to a lifelong process of becoming more culturally competent. Effective cross-cultural communication is a crucial aspect of cultural competence. Nurses need to acknowledge the barriers that can cause cultural misunderstandings and interfere with safe and quality care, and to gain skill in the strategies that promote respectful, patient-centered, cross-cultural communication and culturally congruent care.

Case Study Resolution

Several judgments and actions by the nurse interfered with the provision of effective cross-cultural communication and safe, high-quality nursing care. First, contrary to federal and Joint Commission guidelines, the nurse used a minor child as the interpreter. The child lacked an understanding of medical terminology both in English and in Spanish. The patient who was pregnant (her son did not know) felt embarrassed about discussing female anatomy and reproductive issues with her son, and was unsure if he knew or understood the correct vocabulary. Therefore she referred to her uterine contractions and cramping as stomach pain and did not disclose that she had experienced some bloody spotting. The nurse displayed her frustration and what the patient perceived as disrespect in her facial expression, posture, and behavior, though not in words (patient comes from a high-context culture). The nurse addressed the patient by her first name (did not use a more formal approach such as Ms. or Mrs.), and then essentially ignored her and interacted with her son, facing him and not the patient. The patient felt that the nurse was cold and uncaring, did not demonstrate any concern for her as a person, performed tasks without explaining them, did not evaluate her pain, and did not provide any comfort measures (such as holding her hand or soothing her brow). The patient felt that she was "pushed out the door," with no resolution to her problem. Thus, even when the bleeding continued and worsened, she delayed returning to the hospital because she believed that the nurses and doctors would minimize her symptoms and treat her with disrespect.

When her husband returned home from work and realized her distress, he insisted that she return to the hospital. This time a different nurse made arrangements for the assistance of a trained interpreter. The nurse addressed the patient using a formal title, positioned the interpreter so that she could face the patient, and used facial expressions, eye contact, posture, and touch that conveyed respect and empathy to the patient. Also, she had the interpreter ask the patient if she had any objection to having her husband present and if medical information should be shared with him. Once it was determined that the patient was having a miscarriage and this fact was explained to the patient and her husband in a caring manner, the patient's and husband's responses were emotive. The nurse's verbal (through the interpreter) and nonverbal communication expressed sincere sadness and concern for the couple. She asked if they wanted privacy, if any other family members should be contacted, and eventually asked if there were any cultural or religious beliefs or practices that the nurse could support. Although the outcome was sad for the couple, the patient felt that the care that she received was respectful, supportive, and culturally acceptable. The miscarriage may not have been avoidable, but the patient received inadequate care and prolonged suffering due to the first nurse's lack of cultural and linguistic competence.

Evidence-Based Article

Carnevale, F. A., Vissandjee, B., Nyland, A., & Vinet-Bonn, A. (2009). Ethical considerations in cross-linguistic nursing. *Nursing Ethics, 16*(6), 813–826.

This article presents a narrative review of the empirical evidence of communication barriers encountered during cross-linguistic nursing care, which can perpetuate discrimination and suboptimal care. Using the codes of ethics of the American Nurses Association, the Canadian Nurses Association, and the International Council of Nurses, the authors provide a comparative analysis of the ethical norms within those documents that are relevant to cross-linguistic nursing care. Findings from the comparative analysis include five major ethical norms that are germane to cross-linguistic nursing care: (1) respect for the patient as a unique person; (2) respect for the patient's right to self-determination; (3) respect for patient privacy and confidentiality; (4) responsibility for one's own (nurse's) competence, judgment, and action; and (5) responsibility to promote action that more effectively meets the needs of vulnerable patients, families, and groups. The authors identify implications for nursing education, practice, and research in addressing the ethical challenges encountered within cross-linguistic nursing care.

References

American Association of Colleges of Nursing. (2008). *Cultural competency in baccalaureate nursing education.* Washington, DC: Author.

Ardoin, K. B. & Wilson, K. B. (2010). Cultural diversity: What role does it play in patient safety? *Nursing for Women's Health, 14*(4), 322–326.

Baldwin, D. M. (2003). Disparities in health and health care: Focusing efforts to eliminate unequal burdens. *Online Journal of Nursing Issues, 8*(1). Retrieved from http://gm6.nursingworld.org/MainMenuCategories/ANAMarketplace/ANAPeriodicals/OJIN/TableofContents/Volume82003/No1Jan2003/DisparitiesinHealthandHealthCare.html

Berlin, E., & Fowkes, W. (1983). A teaching framework for cross-cultural health care. *Western Journal of Medicine, 139*, 934–938.

Betancourt, J., Green, A., Carrillo, J., & Ananeh-Firempong, O. (2003). Defining cultural competence: A practical framework for addressing racial/ethnic disparities in health care. *Public Health Reports, 118*, 293–302.

Calvillo, E., Clark, L., Ballantyne, J. E., Pacquiao, D., Purnell, L. D., &Villarruel, A. M. (2009). Cultural competency in baccalaureate nursing education. *Journal of Transcultural Nursing, 20*, 137–145.

Campinha-Bacote, J. (2002). The process of cultural competence in the delivery of healthcare services: A model of care. *Journal of Transcultural Nursing, 13*(3), 181–184.

Cioffi, J. (2003). Communicating with culturally and linguistically diverse patients in an acute care setting: Nurses' experiences. *International Journal of Nursing Studies, 40*, 299–306.

Douglas, M. K., Uhl Pierce, J., Rosenkoetter, M., Pacquiao, D., Clark Callister, L., Hattar-Pollara, M, ..., Purnell, L. (2011). Standards of practice for culturally competent nursing care: 2011 update. *Journal of Transcultural Nursing, 22*(4), 317–333.

Flores, G., Laws, B., Mayo, S., Zuckerman, B., Abreu, M., Medina, L., & Hardt, E. (2003). Errors in medical interpretation and their potential clinical consequences in pediatric encounters. *Pediatrics, 111*(1), 6–14.

Hall, E. (1976). *Beyond culture*. New York: Random House.

Health Resources and Services Administration. (2008). National sample survey of registered nurses. Retrieved from http://datawarehouse.hrsa.gov/nursingsurvey.aspx

Jacobs, E. A., Lauderdale, D. S., Meltzer, D., Shorey, J. M., Levinson, W., & Thisted, R. A. (2001). Impact of interpreter services on delivery of health care to limited-English-proficient patients. *Journal of General Internal Medicine, 16*, 468–474.

Jirwe, M., Gerrish, K., & Emami, A., (2010). Student nurses' experiences of communication in cross-cultural care encounters. *Scandinavian Journal of Caring Sciences, 24*, 436–444.

Joint Commission. (2010). *Advancing effective communication, cultural competence, and patient- and family-centered care: A roadmap for hospitals*. Oakbrook Terrace, IL: Author. Retrieved from http://www.jointcommission.org/assets/1/6/ARoadmapforHospitals finalversion727.pdf

Kleinman, A., Eisenberg, L., & Good, B. (1978). Culture, illness, and care: Clinical lessons from anthropological and cross-cultural research. *Annals of Internal Medicine, 88*(2), 251–258.

Rivadeneyra, R., Elderkin-Thompson, V., Silver, R. C., & Waitzkin, H. (2000). Patient centered-ness in medical encounters requiring an interpreter. *American Journal of Medicine, 108*(6), 470–474.

Smedley, B. D., Stith, A. Y., & Nelson, A. R. (Eds.). (2002). *Unequal treatment: Confronting racial and ethnic disparities in health care*. Washington, DC: National Academic Press.

Tervalon, M., & Murray-Garcia, J. (1998). Cultural humility versus cultural competence: A critical distinction in defining physician training outcomes in multicultural education. *Journal of Health Care for the Poor and Underserved, 9*(2), 117–125.

U.S. Census Bureau. (2010). Overview of race and Hispanic origin 2010: 2010 census briefs. Retrieved from http://www.census.gov/prod/cen2010/briefs/c2010br-02.pdf

The Nurse–Patient Relationship

CHAPTER FIVE

Establishing a Therapeutic Relationship

Lisa Kennedy Sheldon

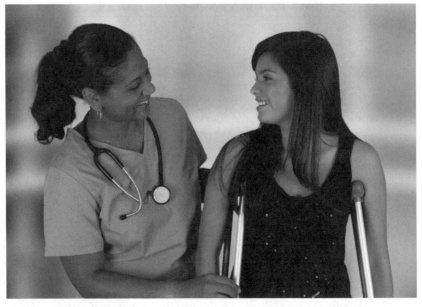

■ CASE STUDY

Susan R. is a 38-year-old woman coming into the outpatient surgery center for a breast biopsy. She sits in the waiting room with her husband and is obviously nervous—staring unblinking at the wall, tapping her feet, and wringing a tissue in her hand. The perioperative nurse approaches Susan to introduce herself and bring her into the operation suite to prepare for surgery.

> *Nurse*: "Mrs. R., I am Laurie Snow, and I will be the nurse working with you today. What do you like to be called?"
>
> *Patient*: "Hello. Call me Sue; that's what everyone else calls me. This is my husband, Andrew."
>
> *Nurse*: (She shakes hands with the patient and her husband.) "It's nice to meet both of you. Sue, I would like to explain what's going to happen today, get a little more information from you, and answer any questions that you may have about the surgery."
>
> *Patient*: "Oh, thank you. I am so scared. I don't know how I am going to get through this."
>
> *Nurse*: "It's common to feel nervous about surgery. My goal is to help you through today. I will explain everything as we go along and answer any questions you and Andrew may have."
>
> *Patient*: "I am glad that you will be there. May my husband come with me?"
>
> *Nurse*: "Of course."

Introduction

In a few moments, the perioperative nurse in the case study has accomplished a great deal toward creating a solid nurse–patient relationship. What did she do?

1. Identified herself by name.
2. Established her credentials and her role.
3. Greeted the patient by her preferred name.
4. Addressed both the patient and her husband by their preferred names.
5. Reflected and normalized the patient's response to the surgery.
6. Offered her assistance in relieving the patient's anxiety by explaining her role.
7. Acknowledged that the patient might have questions and she was there to help.

Good communication skills make the difference between average and excellent nursing care. The therapeutic relationship between the patient and the nurse forms the foundation of nursing care throughout the spectrum of health, illness, healing, and recovery. Some nurse–patient relationships, such as the one in this example, last only a few hours; others, however, may last days, months, or even years. What is exciting about each relationship is how unique and enriching it can be for both the patient and the nurse.

The underlying principles of the therapeutic relationship are the same regardless of the length of the contact: respect, genuineness, empathy, active listening, trust, and confidentiality. The purpose of the therapeutic relationship is to support the patient, to promote healing, and to support or enhance functioning. A therapeutic relationship differs from a social relationship in that it is health focused and patient centered with defined boundaries. Peplau (1991) described the nurse's focused interest in the patient as "professional closeness."

Communication is the cornerstone of the nurse–patient relationship. The focus of communication in the nurse–patient relationship is the patient's needs—that is, patient-centered care. To meet these needs, the nurse must take into consideration multiple factors, including the patient's physical condition, emotional state, cultural preferences, values, needs, readiness to communicate, and ways of relating to others. The timing of communication is also important when working with patients. For example, teaching about a low-cholesterol diet and aerobic exercise is not appropriate during the acute phase of a myocardial infarction. The patient is not in the appropriate physical or emotional state to absorb this information regardless of its importance for overall cardiovascular health. Later, when the patient is preparing for discharge, the nurse may begin teaching about health-promoting behaviors, such as diet and exercise.

Respect: Unconditional Positive Regard

Carl Rogers, in his seminal book published in 1961, defined respect or *unconditional positive regard* as the ability to accept another person's beliefs despite your own personal feelings. Each patient's response to health or illness is a personal way of adapting to challenges. Each patient brings a lifetime of responding and coping with changes, requiring the nurse to be nonjudgmental. Each patient requires respect and acceptance as a unique human being. Acceptance does not mean approval or agreement; rather, it is a nonjudgmental attitude about the patient as a whole person. The goal is to make the patient feel comfortable and legitimize his or her feelings. For example, the nurse might not

---

Box 5-1 Ways to Show Respect

- Introduce yourself by name and professional status and wear a name tag.
- Ask patients what they like to be called. Always begin with the formal (e.g., Mr., Ms., Mrs.), and then use the preferred name.
- Arrange for patient comfort, modesty, and privacy at all times.
- Prepare patients before doing any procedures, particularly those that involve personal space or discomfort.
- Communicate with patients in ways that demonstrate a desire to listen, understand, and help.

---

always understand why patients become angry but acknowledges that they usually have reasons, based on their beliefs and backgrounds, for these emotional responses. Some patients might have unhealthy habits, such as smoking or excessive drinking, that they will not change despite the nurse's best efforts at teaching health-promoting behaviors. Some patients might have difficulty maintaining their personal hygiene. The nurse's goal is to respectfully take into account the patient's symptoms, feelings, values, and beliefs, and to work with the patient to develop the goals of care (Box 5-1). Nurses demonstrate unconditional positive regard by accepting people without negatively judging their basic worth.

Genuineness

The ability to be oneself within the context of a professional role is called *genuineness*. Rogers described genuineness as *congruence*, the willingness to be open and genuine and not hide behind a professional façade. For example, as nurses develop into experts over many clinical experiences, their professional selves come into agreement with their personal selves. As a new nurse, this evolution may not be easy, especially when first starting in the clinical setting. In addition, the nurse will encounter many new patients, some with values and behaviors that the nurse does not accept or even understand. Holding back these judgments may seem less than genuine, yet there are many parts of the personal self that can be shared during nurse–patient interactions that demonstrate true concern for the patient. Genuineness is a welcome part of working in health care because it allows the incorporation of shared humanity and authenticity into nursing care.

Here's an example of a nurse expressing genuineness and care while talking with a patient who has been trying to quit smoking:

> *Patient*: "I have some bad news. After our last appointment, I started smoking again. I tried, really tried, but everyone at home was smoking."
>
> *Nurse*: "I am glad that you tried to quit. It's tough, isn't it? Often, people try to quit many times before succeeding. The more attempts you make to stop smoking, the more likely you will succeed. Let's talk about other strategies. Where can your family smoke that is away from you?"

In this short interchange, the nurse has acknowledged the patient's efforts and the difficulties involved in quitting smoking, offered encouragement, and started working with the patient to solve some of the barriers to stopping smoking.

Another way to be genuine is to show interest in the patient during daily nursing care. As time allows, ask about the patient's family, work, hobbies, or other interests. Older patients often enjoy sharing life experiences and may tell stories about important or funny events in their lives. This is not just superficial chatter. Such information allows you to understand the patient's life, priorities, and previous adjustments to challenges during the current change in health status. Encouraging patients to share their life stories shows interest in them as people and not just as diagnoses or procedures. Sometimes, these stories and experiences can be used when teaching new information.

Genuineness, even as a student or new nurse, is freeing. The first time a student experiences a conflict in congruence might be when introducing himself or herself as a student to a patient. Although it might feel difficult, student nurses should introduce themselves as students, reaffirming that although their knowledge may be limited, their interest in each patient is not. Most patients actually enjoy having a student nurse who has time to give them more attention. Even practicing nurses will have occasions when their time, knowledge, or abilities are limited. Revealing these constraints to patients does not make them "bad" nurses but rather honest ones. As long as limitations are presented with assurances of ongoing interest in the patents' needs, patients are usually understanding and may even try to be helpful.

Nurses may genuinely express some of their feelings with patients within the therapeutic relationship. For example, laughing when a patient brings in a joke

The nurse-patient relationship allows the patient to feel comfortable sharing personal information about his or her health and wellness.

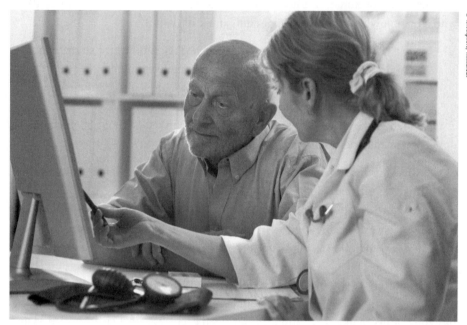

© iStockphoto/Thinkstock

from the Internet that is appropriate and funny can be a bonding experience (see the *Humor* chapter for more on this topic). Likewise, nurses can express sympathy when patients or families are grieving lost loved ones. Using one's own personality when talking with patients humanizes the experience for patients and brings joy to the nurse's work.

Empathy

Nursing is often described as providing empathetic or compassionate care to patients. Four terms are frequently used to describe the emotional work of nursing: altruism, sympathy, compassion, and empathy.

Altruism is defined as (1) understanding the experience of another involving self-sacrifice or (2) unselfish regard and/or devotion to others. Continuing self-sacrifice by nurses may lead to emotional exhaustion and burnout (Henderson, 2001).

Sympathy is the fact or power of sharing the feelings of another and actually experiencing what another person is feeling. Sympathy may actually impair the nurse's ability to care for the patient because the nurse's emotional experience may cloud professional judgment.

Compassion is a feeling of deep sympathy or desire to understand another's experience accompanied by a desire to relieve suffering. Patient suffering may include physical symptoms such as pain, nausea, and shortness of breath; psychological symptoms such as mood, coping, and relationship issues; social problems such as family concerns, community, and financial issues; and problems within the spiritual realm such as faith and finding meaning and closure. Compassionate caring is often included in descriptions of nursing services.

Empathy is educated compassion or the intellectual understanding of the emotional state of another person. It can be described as the nurse's desire to understand what a patient is experiencing from the patient's perspective. Empathy allows nurses the ability to actually see the world from the patient's point of view without experiencing the emotional content. This intellectual understanding allows the nurse to identify the patient's concerns more clearly and intervene more specifically.

Nurses incorporate an empathetic desire to understand the patient's experience combined with a compassionate goal to alleviate suffering. There is probably a spectrum of professional empathy and compassion in nursing. While newer nurses may have a greater desire to understand the experiences of their patients, more experienced nurses tend to use their empathetic desires more efficiently to assess and understand the patient's experience, define the patient's needs, set goals with the patient, deliver appropriate interventions, and assess patient outcomes.

Trust

The establishment of trust is the foundation of all interpersonal relationships and is vitally important to the development of the therapeutic relationship in nursing. In psychoanalytic theories such as that developed by Freud, the development of a sense of trust is a primal need of all human beings (see the chapter titled *The Nurse as a Person: Theories of Self and Nursing*). On the physical, emotional, and spiritual levels, trust is essential when patients are placed in a vulnerable position in healthcare settings. Patients need to believe that nurses are honest, knowledgeable, dependable, and accepting of who they are as people. Erikson (1963) described trust as the reliance on consistency, sameness, and continuity of experiences provided by familiar and predictable things and people. Trust is a choice that a person makes, based on the need to trust others. Nurses can facilitate the process of developing trust in their patients with the behaviors described in Box 5-2.

Box 5-2	Facilitating Trust

- Listen carefully; patients will feel understood and cared for.
- Treat patients respectfully; patients will feel like valuable human beings.
- Be honest and consistent; patients will feel that nurses are trustworthy.
- Follow through on commitments; patients will feel that their care is predictable and dependable.
- Have an accepting attitude; patients will be more comfortable sharing information about themselves.

Confidentiality

Nurses have moral and legal obligations not to share patient information with others, except in specific circumstances. Beyond the dictates of legal statutes, it is important from the standpoint of trust that patients know that their personal information will be kept confidential. Patients will be more forthcoming and honest in their revelations and responses if they feel that their information is confidential. Nurses should arrange for privacy in the physical setting before discussing sensitive information with patients. Providing privacy may include finding an empty room or asking an ambulatory roommate to leave the room or closing a door.

Keeping patient information confidential includes not speaking in public places where information could be overheard, such as elevators and cafeterias. It also includes confidentiality with electronic information. Nurse–patient confidentiality can be breached only for the following reasons:

- Suspicion of abuse of minors or elders
- Commission of a crime
- Threat or potential threat of harm to oneself or others

For more on confidentiality, see the *Patients as People: Standards to Guide Communication* chapter.

The Nurse–Patient Relationship

The establishment of the nurse–patient relationship is a conscious commitment on the part of the nurse to care for a patient. It also symbolizes an agreement between the nurse and the patient to work together for the good of the patient.

While the nurse accepts primary responsibility for setting the structure and purpose of the relationship, the nurse uses a patient-centered approach to develop the relationship and meet the patient's needs. The nurse functions within professional, legal, ethical, and personal boundaries as described in the chapter titled *The Nurse as a Person: Theories of Self and Nursing.* The nurse also respects the uniqueness of each patient and strives to understand his or her response to changes in health. Nurses establish relationships with patients by integrating the concepts of respect, empathy, trust, genuineness, and confidentiality into their interactions.

One of the earliest nursing theorists to explore the nurse–patient relationship and nursing communication was Hildegard Peplau (1952, 1991, 1992, 1997). Peplau developed a landmark theory, the theory of interpersonal relations, which emphasizes reciprocity in the interpersonal relationship between the nurse and the patient. Peplau's theory moved thinking about nursing from what nurses do *to* patients to thinking about what nurses do *with* patients, thereby envisioning nursing as an interactive and collaborative process between the nurse and the patient.

Peplau identified five phases of the nurse–patient relationship: orientation, identification, exploitation, resolution, and termination. In Peplau's theory of interpersonal relations, these phases are therapeutic and focus on interpersonal interactions.

1. Orientation: The patient seeks help, and the nurse assists the patient to identify the problem and the extent of help needed.
2. Identification: The patient relates to the nurse from an independent, dependent, or interdependent posture, and the nurse assures the patient that he or she understands the meaning of his or her situation.
3. Exploitation: The patient uses the nurse's services and other resources on the basis of his or her needs.
4. Resolution: The patient's old needs are resolved, and more mature goals emerge.
5. Termination: The patient and the nurse evaluate the progress of the interventions toward the intended goals, review their time together and end the relationship.

Orientation Phase

Beginning the nurse–patient relationship requires unique communication skills. Every day people communicate with those around them by listening, talking, sharing, laughing, reassuring, and caring. Nurses use these basic components of communication to establish a helping relationship. Although different from the other relationships in life such as friendships, family roles, casual contacts, community relationships, and professional alliances, relationships between nurses and patients are still a connection between people. Particular communication skills are effective for nurses when they begin these unique relationships with patients.

As described by Peplau, the relationship formally begins during the orientation phase. The nurse sets the tone for the relationship by greeting the patient properly: "I am Laurie Snow and I will be the nurse taking care of you during the day today." The nurse in the case study introduced herself by name and professional status. The tone and warmth of the words during this exchange can promote connectedness between the nurse and the patient. Often a handshake is an appropriate component of the introduction, but this will vary by cultural setting and acuity of the clinical situation. Patients are addressed by their formal names first and then asked what they prefer to be called. Establishing rapport might begin with talking about clinically relevant topics, such as health issues and concerns, or it may begin with more social discourse about the weather, parking, or office surroundings. Patients begin interacting in their usual patterns, and nurses both direct and follow the patients' comments to establish rapport and trust. Nurses foster trust by being consistent in both their words and actions. This consistency conveys dependability and competence. The orientation phase is important in developing a foundation for the therapeutic relationship.

After the greeting phase, the nurse clarifies the purpose and nature of the relationship. This includes providing information about the appointment or interview, describing the nurse's role, helping the patient provide pertinent information, and describing the goals of the relationship. Each nurse has a personal style, so the delivery of this information will vary by person. It is important not to overlook this part of the relationship as a superficial aspect of the "real work." Establishing the purpose and goals of the relationship is fundamental not only to the delivery of care but also to the evaluation of the relationship and outcomes during the termination phase. Also, anxiety levels decrease when the patient knows what to expect and participates in the establishment of the relationship. The nurse seeks to promote trust and reduce anxiety by being genuine, respectful, and informative. Receptive body language and active listening help patients feel more comfortable and remain focused during the next phase.

Data collection also occurs during the orientation phase. Collecting data for the nursing assessment requires active participation from the patient to identify health status and functioning. The nurse needs an open mind to understand the patient's perception of the problem(s) and the need for treatment. What might seem apparent to the nurse may not be the patient's view of the situation. For example, the nurse could begin with a general question, "What brought you into the hospital today?" or "What kind of assistance can we provide for you?" While more specific questions on the nursing assessment might provide a focus for the initial data collection, it is important for the nurse to take the time to listen—really hear—the patient's needs and expectations. This prevents disappointment during and at the end of the relationship if care did not proceed as the patient anticipated. The nurse can correct misinformation and clarify the situation before actual interventions begin.

The orientation phase ends with a therapeutic contract. While not usually a formal document, the verbal contract explains the roles of the nurse and patient and the goals of the relationship. From the case study, the nurse concludes the initial meeting with the patient by saying, "Sue, I will be with you during your breast biopsy, from now until you go home. I will start with a brief questionnaire. Then I will explain what will happen today. Before I begin, do you have any other questions at this time?"

Identification Phase

The working segment of the relationship begins with the identification phase. The nurse and patient work together to identify problems and set specific problem-oriented goals. Health problems are identified during data collection, and appropriate interventions are developed in the nursing care plan. Mutual goal setting allows patients to be active participants in their care. Nurses can also help patients explore feelings about their situation, including fear, anxiety, and helplessness, and direct their energies toward actions. Identification of personal strengths and resources may help patients cope with the current health problems and actively participate in their care. In the case study, the patient later expressed fear about pain during the breast biopsy. The nurse said, "Sue, you are concerned about pain during the breast biopsy. I will talk with the surgeon about medications during the procedure. I will also be with you during the biopsy in case you have any questions or you begin to feel uncomfortable."

Exploitation Phase

During the exploitation phase, the nurse assists the patient in using health services. The active work of the relationship happens during exploitation. Interventions appropriate to the mutually planned goals are carried out with ongoing reassessment and reevaluation. Sometimes, even well-planned interventions need to be reviewed, and new, more realistic goals need to be established. The therapeutic relationship allows the nurse and patient to work together during the exploitation phase. The patient uses identified strengths and resources to regain control and develop solutions.

Resolution Phase

Ending a therapeutic relationship requires a period of resolution that Peplau aptly named the resolution phase. Some of the most satisfying parts of a nurse's job are caring relationships with patients. Often, very meaningful sharing has taken place between the patient and the nurse during some challenging times. The relationship was originally established with a purpose and, frequently, a time frame. For example, the perioperative nurse at an outpatient surgical center has a short time frame for the relationship with the patient who is undergoing arthroscopy. In contrast, the oncology nurse has a long-term relationship with the patient with recurrent colon cancer that might end with the patient dying. Each relationship, both the short-term and the long-term partnership, requires preparation for the end or resolution.

Termination Phase

Endings are a time for review and growth. The termination phase is often overlooked because of the emphasis in health care on diagnosis and treatment. The ending of the therapeutic relationship, no matter how brief, can be a valuable time for the patient and the nurse to examine the achievement of their goals and review their time together. The nurse uses summarization skills to evaluate the progress of the interventions toward the intended goals. This review can bring a sense of accomplishment and closure for both parties.

Emotions are part of ending relationships. Caring attitudes and shared experiences, especially in long-term relationships, may result in sadness and ambivalence at the end of a nurse–patient relationship. Termination of a relationship can awaken feelings of loss from previous relationships. Acknowledgment of the feelings that arise is helpful in dissipating sadness and learning healthy skills for dealing with endings and loss. The termination phase is also the time when unmet goals are identified by the nurse and patient that may require referral and follow-up care.

Patients and nurses respond in a variety of ways to ending relationships. Each brings his or her prior experiences of endings and losses and often some ambivalent feelings. When the end is approaching, patients might regress, become anxious, act more superficially with the nurse, or become more dependent. The nurse might detach, spending less time with the patient in preparation for termination of the relationship. Any and all of these responses are within the realm of normal. As the end becomes inevitable, the nurse and the patient might even develop feelings of anger and/or abandonment. Nurses and patients can and should talk about ending their relationship, taking time to reminisce about the goals accomplished, the moments shared, and even the sadness at ending the relationship if that is the case. All these feelings are normal responses to the ending of a relationship, even a professional one. Nurses should not avoid the discomfort they feel during these discussions because the relationship was well worth the time. The therapeutic relationship between the nurse and patient will finish with a completeness and satisfaction that is rewarding for both the nurse and the patient.

Setting Boundaries

When establishing the nurse–patient relationship, the purpose and goals of the relationship are set by certain social parameters. Boundaries are important, both legally and ethically, and help to establish the roles of the nurse and the patient, including the nature of the relationship. This therapeutic relationship is a professional relationship revolving around the patient's needs. Objectivity is an important attribute when assessing the patient's needs and providing competent and professional care. Being a compassionate nurse means using an empathetic approach but not being so emotionally close to a patient that impaired objectivity and judgment compromise patient care. Setting boundaries for appropriate topics and conversations allows nurses to effectively function in their roles.

Some specific strategies for maintaining professional boundaries include the following:

- Clearly define the roles in the relationship and who can participate.
- Establish clear boundaries between yourself and others.

- Recognize that different cultures and ethnic groups may have varying rules for interactions.
- Develop self-awareness regarding your responses to the needs of others.

Self-awareness allows nurses to understand which emotions, responses, and needs are their own and which are the needs of others. It also allows nurses to recognize the signs of emotional exhaustion, burnout, and over-involvement with patients and find ways to ventilate and rejuvenate themselves. Self-awareness fosters a balanced use of the professional and personal selves, thereby establishing congruence in the professional role.

For example, Bob is a nurse in an outpatient internal medicine practice who has been working with an elderly woman, Mrs. R., for the last 5 years. He has cared for Mrs. R. during many stressful episodes of angina and has also been involved in her life during the recent loss of her husband at the local hospice house. This patient even reminds the nurse of his grandmother. One day, Bob observes Mrs. R. being given advice by another nurse in the office with which he does not agree. Rather than wait for a private moment to discuss the issue with his coworker, he interrupts the conversation, corrects the other nurse in front of Mrs. R., and gives the patient what he feels is better advice. This episode breached at least two tenets of good communication. First, a nurse should not correct a coworker in front of a patient; such an action is disrespectful to the coworker. Second, this encounter may make the patient feel that some workers in the office may not be competent, creating worry and distrust. Perhaps Bob felt possessive or concerned about Mrs. R.'s care beyond the level of professionalism and objectivity. Caring for patients can often blur the boundaries between professional behavior and emotional responses. Through self-awareness, the nurse would have been better able to differentiate between compassionate care and over-involvement with a patient that endangers the ability to provide competent, professional, collegial, and objective care.

Self-Disclosure

Self-disclosure is a tricky topic for many students and even practicing nurses. While they want to appear professional and not divulge personal details or feelings, they often find themselves being asked personal questions by patients. Professors often encourage students to keep the focus of interactions on the patients and their needs. The reality of nurse–patient relationships is often more complex, however, and nurses may be at a loss to firmly define personal and professional boundaries. Spontaneous questions during routine care require nurses to respond sincerely. When is self-disclosure appropriate, and how much personal information should a nurse reveal?

Patients might ask questions about personal details about the nurse, such as "Where are you from?" or "Do you have any children?" These questions might be used by patients to find common ground for conversation or to make them more comfortable with their revelation of personal details. Whatever the reason, both students and practicing nurses need to establish, first, that the patient is the focus of their time together. Then, as time or the relationship permits, the sharing of other information may be appropriate. However, intimate details about the nurse are never shared with the patient. When in doubt, the nurse should ask another trusted colleague, practicing nurse, or professor about a particular patient question prior to responding. It is always within the nurse's bounds to say, "I don't think that question is relevant to your care. Let's focus on you ..."

Summary

The nurse–patient relationship is the cornerstone of nursing care throughout the spectrum of health, illness, and recovery. The establishment of this relationship is facilitated by the nurse and is patient centered and goal oriented. While some aspects of this relationship follow predictable steps, other parts may be complicated by patient expectations and the intricacies of interpersonal communication. Awareness of the nurse's role sets the boundaries of the relationship, but within these bounds are limitless possibilities for communication that may be both therapeutic and enriching for both parties.

Case Study Resolution

The nurse, Laurie, stayed with Sue throughout the breast biopsy and recovery. While Sue was recovering from her sedation, Laurie went to the waiting room to talk with Andrew to let him know that Sue was finished with the procedure and doing well. When Sue was ready for discharge, Laurie spoke with both her and her husband to explain the discharge instructions and follow-up care. The couple seemed relieved to have the procedure over and were anxious about the pathology results. Laurie gave them her name and phone number in case they had any questions once they returned home.

EXERCISES

ESTABLISHING THE RELATIONSHIP

Break into groups of three, with one person assuming the role of the "patient," one the "nurse," and one the "observer."

- "Nurse": Establish the relationship.
- "Patient": Assume the role in the scenario.
- "Observer": Give feedback on the establishment of the nurse–patient relationship and the verbal and nonverbal communication.

Take turns playing each role with the three following scenarios.

1. The patient is a 20-year-old single mother who is bringing her 2-month-old baby in for a series of immunizations. The nurse works full time in the pediatricians' office but not always with the same pediatrician.
2. The patient is a 38-year-old male arriving in the ambulatory surgical center for an arthroscopy. The nurse will be with the patient both preoperatively and postoperatively.
3. The patient is a 28-year-old woman, grava 1 para 0, arriving in the maternity ward in early labor. The nurse will be with the patient during this shift and tomorrow on the evening shift.

Evidence-Based Article

Belcher, M., & Jones, L. K. (2009). Graduate nurses experiences of developing trust in the nurse–patient relationship. *Contemporary Nurse, 31*(2), 142–152.

In this qualitative study, seven new graduate nurses were interviewed about their experiences developing trust in nurse–patient relationships. The nurses described rapport as needing to be developed before trust can be established in these relationships. The authors recommend teaching communication skills to increase rapport and the identification of effective strategies to provide care when rapport is not achieved in the relationship.

References

Erikson, E. (1963). *Childhood and society*. New York: Norton.

Henderson, A. (2001). Emotional labor and nursing: An underappreciated aspect of caring work. *Nursing Inquiry, 8*(2), 130–138.

Peplau, H. E. (1952). *Interpersonal relations in nursing*. New York: Putnam.

Peplau, H. E. (1991). *Interpersonal relations in nursing*. New York: Springer.

Peplau, H. (1992). Interpersonal relations: A theoretical framework for application in practice. *Nursing Science Quarterly, 5*(1), 13–18.

Peplau, H. E. (1997). Peplau's theory of interpersonal relations. *Nursing Science Quarterly, 10*(4), 162–167.

Rogers, C. (1961). *On becoming a person*. Boston: Houghton Mifflin.

CHAPTER SIX

Interviewing Skills:
A Clinical Art and Science

Lisa Kennedy Sheldon

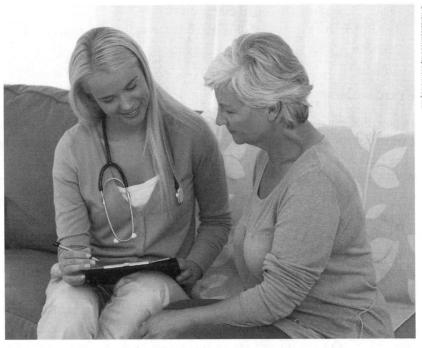

■ Case Study

Mrs. S., a 57-year-old Hispanic woman complaining of chest pain, is brought to the emergency room by her adult children. Her children say that she has been very weepy since her husband's death 2 months ago. This morning, she began holding her chest and describing a heaviness in her heart. Mrs. S. says that her heart aches since her husband died, and she does not want to get out of bed in the morning and doesn't care about food. The emergency room nurse begins her assessment.

> *Nurse*: "Hello, Mrs. S. I am Laurie Gardner, and I am the nurse who will be taking care of you. How are you feeling tonight?"
>
> *Mrs. S.*: "Not good. I am so sad without my husband." (She is weeping and holding a tissue to her chest.)
>
> *Nurse*: "I am sorry for your loss. You are holding your chest. Do you have pain in your chest?"
>
> *Mrs. S.*: "My heart aches but it feels better when I stop and sit still."
>
> *Nurse*: "Does anything else hurt?"
>
> *Mrs. S.*: "My neck aches sometimes, and my stomach feels bad."
>
> *Nurse*: "How long have you had these problems?"
>
> *Mrs. S.*: "Since my husband died, but I feel worse since I raked the lawn this morning."

Introduction

How does this emergency room nurse begin to sift through the patient's symptoms and responses? Not only do patients present with health issues, but they also bring to each encounter their own interpretations of their health status. They arrive in the healthcare setting with their own cultural beliefs and values that may affect their perception of health or illness. Sometimes they may have emotional and physical symptoms that overlap. Although the science of nursing and communication may direct the patient assessment, it is the art of nursing that derives the meaning from the patient's words. Interviewing skills are essential to understanding patients' health and concerns to arrive at accurate conclusions and begin effective interventions.

As discussed in the *Establishing a Therapeutic Relationship* chapter, therapeutic relationships are based on trust, empathy, and respect. The establishment of trust is particularly important when obtaining personal information from patients because they are more apt to share their feelings and symptoms when they trust the nurse. Empathy allows nurses to try to see the situation from their patients' perspectives. Respect for the patient creates a nonjudgmental view of the patient and his or her attitudes, values, and feelings. This chapter reviews interviewing skills that produce accurate, reliable, and complete information about each patient to direct appropriate and effective nursing interventions.

Setting Goals

Every encounter between a patient and a nurse begins with the establishment of the roles each will play during the encounter. Nurses have roles that are both professionally and culturally defined. As discussed in the *Patients as People: Standards to Guide Communication* chapter, nurses must adhere to standards and guidelines set by nursing organizations, laws, and the institutions and organizations where they are employed. Patients also bring expectations about the nurse's role based on public information, social anecdotes, images in the media, and even personal experiences. Patients may also have their own agenda or problems they believe nurses and other healthcare providers may be able to improve with appropriate health care. Establishing the guidelines early in the relationship will make the encounter more predictable and less stressful for the patient and more productive for both the nurse and the patient (see Fortin, Dwamena, Framkel, & Smith, 2012; p. 30, Figure 3-1). Nurses also have expectations of patients and how they will participate in their care.

Becoming a patient is a curious and often dehumanizing experience. First, a person walks in the door of a hospital or healthcare facility and removes his or her clothing, donning the patient uniform (the "johnny"), puts his or her worldly possessions in a bag or behind a door, and leaves behind family and normal surroundings and routines. This experience alone often creates feelings of fear, powerlessness, and dependency in a patient. Yet, as healthcare providers, nurses expect patients to reveal intimate facts about themselves and actively participate in their care while being completely removed from their normal environment and perhaps not feeling well. Not all patients can fulfill these expectations or even understand what is expected from them. It is important for nurses to try to understand the patient's experience, to explain the plan of care, and to work with each patient to set realistic and achievable goals. Nurses can also facilitate the patient's role in decision making by providing explanations of the processes, the proposed interventions, and expected outcomes.

Box 6-1   How to Set Goals

- Define the nurse's role to the patient.
- Explore the patient's needs, concerns, priorities, and abilities.
- Set realistic, measurable, and achievable goals with the patient.
- Ensure that patients understand their care.

Working collaboratively with patients allows for mutual goal setting and the development of more realistic plans (Box 6-1). Collaboration also helps patients take more control of their health and feel more satisfied with their healthcare experiences.

The Role of Student Nurses

Within this discussion of establishing roles is an important role that is often overlooked: the nursing student. While this role may be uncomfortable, nursing students should accurately identify themselves and their role to their patients. On the positive side, many patients feel that they are helping students to learn and they actually enjoy the individual attention provided by student nurses. Students often are less confident in their abilities and knowledge and may be reluctant to reveal their lack of knowledge. All nurses, including students, will not have the answers to all questions asked by patients and their families. Student nurses, in particular, need to answer patient questions sensitively and honestly admit when they are lacking answers and need to seek more information. When nurses or students acknowledge the need for help or seek more information, patients perceive more transparency in the nurse–patient relationship. This transparency, in turn, builds trust in the relationship.

It is important for nurses to project confidence and honesty so that patients feel safe and cared for, and believe they can trust their nurses. Students often ask how they can display confidence when they are still learning and do not know all the answers. Remember—it is possible to be confident both in established skills and in the ability to find information to help patients. Experienced nurses continue to learn and seek answers, even after they have many years of clinical experience.

Active Listening

Active listening is an interactive process between the nurse and the patient—*to understand and to be understood*. Communication is also a process of mutual influence—what the patient and the nurse say influences the other party. Active listening involves the nurse carefully hearing the patient's message, understanding

The establishment of trust is important prior to obtaining personal information from patients.

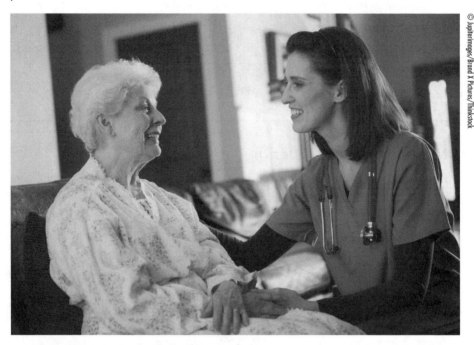

© Jupiterimages/Brand X Pictures/Thinkstock

the meaning of the words, and providing feedback. When patients honestly share their experiences, nurses can better grasp the current health issues for each patient, understand changes in functioning, and explore each patient's responses to changes in health. Listening requires observation to attend to and understand both verbal and nonverbal messages. Compiling as much information as possible allows nurses to identify appropriate goals with their patients.

An important skill for nurses, active listening can be learned with practice (Box 6-2). While it sounds simple, it requires the active suspension of the nurse's other thoughts and feelings and a shift in focus to the content of the patient's message and behavior. Rather than judging or quickly responding with rote phrases such as "I know," the nurse must listen carefully to what patients are saying—or perhaps not saying—about their experience. Identification of the patient's experience directs further questions to completely understand the situation. Nurses should take care to not jump ahead too quickly when patients are quiet, but rather allow the patient to guide the direction of the conversation at a pace that is comfortable. If time constraints interfere, nurses can gently direct the assessment by describing the restrictions on their time to their patients while offering additional opportunities as time permits.

Box 6-2 Body Posture During Active Listening

- Sit upright with torso facing the patient, leaning slightly toward the patient.
- Keep arms and legs relaxed, not crossed.
- Try to sit at eye level, maintaining direct eye contact but not staring. (Note: Direct eye contact is not always culturally appropriate and might require modification.)
- Nod or smile to acknowledge the patient.
- Relax and listen.

Barriers to Active Listening

Many factors can influence the ability of the nurse and patient to communicate effectively. Some factors are recognizable and readily changed, whereas others might necessitate a delay until a more conducive situation arises. The *setting* and *timing* of an interaction, as well as anxiety levels in the patient or nurse, can impede active listening and effective communication. The setting should be private so that the patient feels comfortable divulging personal information. When in doubt, the nurse should ask the patient, "Do you feel comfortable talking here?" or "Where do you want to meet so we can talk?" A private setting also allows for the sharing and protection of confidential information.

The timing of an interaction is very important to therapeutic communication. If the patient is not ready or able to talk, then meaningful conversation may be limited. The nurse should assess the patient's readiness to talk and the timeliness of the topic prior to initiating a dialogue. For example, if a patient has just returned to the hospital unit after a bowel resection and colostomy creation, then teaching about deep breathing would be timely, but a discussion about changing the colostomy bag should wait until later in the recovery process.

Factors such as anxiety may cause difficulties in listening as well as talking for any person. Patients may be nervous about their diagnosis, making it more difficult for them to listen. They might try to "laugh it off" or use silence or sarcasm to avoid exploration of anxiety-producing subjects. Also, the amount of information that a patient can process decreases as his or her anxiety level increases. At other times, information may lower anxiety levels by decreasing uncertainty, such as often happens during preoperative teaching. Useful strategies to reduce anxiety include active listening, honesty, calm behavior, setting limits, pacing the amount of information provided, and encouraging patients to discuss their concerns

(Arnold & Boggs, 2011, pp. 126–128). Therapeutic nursing communication is often an effective intervention to reduce anxiety.

Anxiety can also impair the nurse's ability to listen and engage in more difficult conversations. Some conversations are perceived as more difficult by nurses, such as conversations with angry patients, discussions with patients with metastatic cancer, and even challenging conversations within the nurse–patient–physician triangle (Sheldon, Barrett, & Ellington, 2006). The nurse may also be anxious about a particular new treatment, or the situation itself may be tense, such as during a cardiac arrest. For example, when a patient is acutely ill and physically unstable, an inexperienced nurse may become anxious and not hear the patient describing other symptoms. While there may be no way to decrease tension during certain situations, it is important to realize that listening and judgment can be impeded during anxiety-producing situations. Nurses can turn to one another to confirm what they believe is happening and support one another during stressful situations. Asking for help, expressing anxiety, and timing meaningful conversations are examples of how nurses can support one another and lower anxiety levels.

Silence

While this text focuses mainly on verbal communication, it is also necessary to write about the uses of silence (Box 6-3). It has been said that one cannot hear when talking. Silence can be one of the most potent parts of listening. It allows the importance of a verbal message to sink in and permits adequate time for composing a thoughtful response. Silence after serious conversation conveys the importance of the discussed topic prior to moving on to the next subject. When the patient is silent, it might indicate that a message was powerful or the content provoked strong

---

Box 6-3   Some Uses of Silence

- Allow dissipation of emotion.
- Convey a respectful presence.
- Allow active listening.
- Acknowledge a powerful message.
- Permit careful composition of responses.

Table 6-1 How to Respond to Silence

Possible Reasons for Patient Silence	Nurse Responses
To avoid discussion	Analyze the meaning of silence. Try, "You seem quiet. Would you like to share your thoughts?"
To protect oneself	Provide reassurance if the patient is feeling threatened or anxious.
To avoid disclosure	Reassure the patient that you will keep information confidential. Allow more time for the patient to develop a sense of trust.
To regroup during intense or emotional conversation	Give the patient time to gather himself or herself. Resist the urge to fill the silence with talk.

emotions. Allowing silence to continue after the expression of intense content conveys respect for what the patient has said. Sometimes silence is used by patients to avoid disclosure or to avoid anxiety-producing topics (Table 6-1).

Silences can become too long and uncomfortable for some people—both nurses and patients. Nurses should try to avoid breaking a silence because of their own personal discomfort. With experience, it becomes easier for nurses to sense when a conversation needs restarting or when words of comfort or even a touch may be helpful to the patient.

Types of Responses

Gaining more information requires actively listening to the patient, followed by responding from the nurse. Three types of responses may be useful in gathering accurate data during the assessment: restatement, reflection, and clarification. In these examples, a 71-year-old woman with a history of congestive heart failure arrives in the urgent care department complaining of shortness of breath.

Restatement

Restatement is an initial response that involves paraphrasing what was said. Used sparingly, restatement acknowledges that the listener has heard what was said and is useful when beginning an interview and allows patients to clarify or expand on information.

Patient: "I feel like I can't catch my breath."

Nurse: "It is difficult for you to catch your breath."

Reflection

Reflection involves restating what was said and also reflecting the emotional undertones. This technique is more helpful as the conversation develops.

Patient: "I am scared that my breathing will never get better."

Nurse: "You are worried that we don't have treatments to help your breathing."

Clarification

Clarification utilizes simplification and summarization to make clear, concise statements about the patient's experience.

Patient: "Every day, I try to do my usual housework, but I have to stop and rest after a few minutes. Even getting the newspaper is tiring."

Nurse: "Your breathing makes it difficult to do your normal activities. That must be very frustrating."

Patient: "I don't know what I am going to do. I have tried so many medicines. Is there anything that will make it better?"

Patient-Centered Interviewing

Using careful responses and active listening helps nurses understand the problems at hand and helps patients to express their concerns. Nurses may be perceived as being in control and having more power by patients—a perspective that may impede disclosure (Greene & Burleson, 2003, pp. 921–923). Actively engaging the patient in the interview through the use of accurate assessment of patient verbal and nonverbal behavior and appropriate questions will improve the relationship and the information gathered during the interview. The patient in the previous example is not only having difficulty with the activities of daily living because of her shortness of breath but is also frightened about the future and her treatment options. The nurse's acknowledgment of the emotional content provides support to the patient while clarifying the patient's concerns. Active listening involves hearing not only the facts but also the attached feelings or emotional response. By listening carefully and watching the patient, the nurse demonstrates understanding in multiple ways, such as paying attention and reflecting the content and meaning of the patient's words while continuing to gather information.

Certain responses may be helpful in eliciting more detailed information as well as validating the patient's experience. Helpful ways to respond include interchangeable responses and additive responses (Box 6-4). Conversely, ignoring or minimizing the patient's experience may stunt the assessment, threaten the therapeutic relationship, and curtail meaningful communication (Box 6-5).

Box 6-4   Helpful Ways to Respond

- Interchangeable response: Respond to the patient's feelings by rephrasing his or her concerns at the same level of intensity.
  Patient: "I had so much pain yesterday that I couldn't move. I was so scared."

  Nurse: "Severe pain can be very frightening."
- Additive response: Recognize what the patient is saying and address what may be concerning him or her or offer reassurance.
  Patient: "I tried the pain pills, but even they didn't work."

  Nurse: "You had so much pain that you are afraid that nothing will make it better. We will talk about different ways to make you more comfortable. Let's talk about what makes the pain better or worse."

Box 6-5   Less Helpful Ways to Respond

- Ignoring: Ignoring is either not hearing or acting as though what the patient has said is not understood.
  Patient: "Since the surgery, I have days when the pain is so bad that I cannot get up the stairs."

  Nurse: "How is your appetite?"
- Minimizing: Minimizing is superficially acknowledging what has been said but responding with less intensity than expressed by the patient.
  Patient: "When the pain gets really bad, I just lay on the couch."

  Nurse: "The pain can't be that bad."

Different methods of responding can be used to gather accurate and detailed information during the assessment. In another example, Mr. B., who prefers to be called Pete, is a 28-year-old man who arrives for his annual checkup with multiple vague complaints.

Pete: "I just came for my checkup."

Nurse: "How have you been?"

Pete: "I don't know. I just don't feel very hungry lately. Otherwise, I'm okay."

Nurse: "You don't have much of an appetite. I see that your weight is down 7 pounds this year. When did your appetite change?"

Pete: "It's been going on for months. I just feel nauseous a lot. It got so bad I even tried my mother's medicine."

Nurse: "You took your mother's medicine to help your nausea?"

Pete: "Yes. She has been getting chemotherapy for pancreatic cancer. They gave her medicine for nausea."

Nurse: "Your mother has pancreatic cancer?"

Pete: (Weeping quietly) "She is not doing well. We live together and every day she looks smaller to me. She has no appetite. I don't know what I am going to do."

Nurse: (Placing her hand on Pete's hand) "I am sorry. This must be very difficult for you."

In this situation, the nurse listened carefully to the patient and used helpful and additive responses to reach the source of the patient's problems. Rather than skipping over the patient's first response, the nurse delved deeper into the patient's experience and found that his mother's illness could be contributing to Pete's physical symptoms. Further evaluation and physical assessment would be necessary to completely understand Pete's symptoms, but the nurse wisely listened and learned more about the patient's experience before jumping to conclusions or moving on to the next task.

With clinical experience, nurses can develop flexible communication skills to respond to patients in a variety of ways. Helpful responses elicit more information because they acknowledge the patient's experience. During the previous example, the nurse first tried reflecting or paraphrasing what Pete said with the same level of intensity. The nurse built on the information that he shared by using additive responses. Each response and question was used to validate what Pete had said and build upon prior answers. Also, by reflecting the intensity of Pete's emotions, the nurse acknowledged how Pete was feeling and helped him feel "heard."

The ability to understand patients' concerns, feelings, and symptoms improves with each clinical interaction, honing those communication skills that accurately assess patients as well as provide support and reassurance.

Objectivity

To obtain accurate information during an interview, the nurse must be objective. What is being objective? It means trying to remove one's own beliefs and prejudices from the patient's words and behaviors (Box 6-6). It also means distinguishing between the patient's interpretation and the actual symptoms. While Mrs. S. (from the case study at the beginning of this chapter) is deeply saddened by her husband's death, her chest pain is the first priority for the emergency room nurse. While multiple problems may be present in this case, if the nurse focused only on the sadness and possible depression, then she would miss the possible cardiac origin of the symptoms.

Reliability

Every time patients come into contact with healthcare providers, whether it is a nurse, a physician, or a physical therapist, they have a different experience. They tell their stories and may receive a variety of responses from different providers. Patients filter this information to fit their own interpretations of their health. As an interviewer, the nurse tries to achieve some objective recount of each patient's symptoms that could reliably be obtained again by another provider.

Reliability depends on multiple factors. First, a patient might change his or her story over time, depending on the reactions he or she receives from different

---

Box 6-6   Keys to Objectivity

- Listen to what the patient is saying by being quiet and observing the patient, listening to his or her words and the tone of the message while watching for nonverbal cues. What is not said may be as important as the spoken words.

- Restate what you have heard back to the patient to check for understanding and accuracy.

- Use phrases like "Could you tell me more about . . ." or "I think you said . . . Is this correct?"

- Convey a sincere desire to understand.

providers. Second, each professional has different skills at obtaining information. Finally, different providers might be looking for different information. For example, in the case study at the beginning of the chapter, the physician would look for diagnostic cues (substernal pain on exertion), whereas a physical therapist would gather data about physical functioning (back strain when raking).

What enhances the reliability of information received from a patient? A standardized nursing assessment form is a great place to begin for students or newer nurses. It provides questions that can be used consistently and later customized for individual patients. With time, experienced nurses will detect nuances in the way a patient responds: A pause might mean the patient is unsure of how to respond, or a gesture, such as covering the mouth, perhaps means that the patient is holding back a comment.

Listening also includes looking for nonverbal cues. Nurses may use their intuition based on previous experiences to probe deeper, depending on the situation. The experienced nurse will use observations of verbal and nonverbal cues to phrase the next question in the assessment or to acknowledge how a patient might be feeling.

Styles of Questions

According to Riley (2012), nurses may spend up to half of their time asking patients and families questions. Interviewing patients requires asking questions to gather more detailed information. Most assessment forms collect historical data using a combination of open- and closed-ended questions and menu questions.

Closed-ended questions usually elicit short answers or "yes" or "no" responses. This sort of structured question can be used to gather consistent data. An example of a useful closed-ended question is "Are you allergic to any medicines?"

To obtain a more complete assessment, however, nurses often ask open-ended questions to allow for more informative responses. Open-ended questions are useful in obtaining information about symptoms and feelings. Examples of open-ended questions are "How would you describe your pain?" instead of the closed-end "Do you have any pain?", and "What other surgeries have you had in the past?" instead of the closed-ended "Have you had any other surgeries?"

Menu questions provide a variety of choices for answers. The patient chooses one response, providing another reliable method of collecting information.

At the beginning of an interview, it is useful to start with open-ended questions pertaining to the patient's general status and health history and then move to the specific issues (Box 6-7). The "w/h" questions (who, what, when, where, why,

---

Box 6-7 How to Proceed with an Interview

- Start with general open-ended questions.
- Move to specific open-ended questions.
- Use w/h questions (who, what, when, where, why, how).
- Offer a menu question to help direct the patient.
- Use closed-ended questions to validate the patient's description and then summarize.

---

and how) are open ended and may be used to address specific symptoms. Next, directed or closed-ended questions can provide greater detail about the specific problem. Such questions are useful in gathering factual information and summarizing what has been said. The use of menu questions provides the patient with a variety of answers to choose from.

General Open-Ended Question

Nurse: "What brought you into the emergency room today?"
Patient: "I have been feeling dizzy all day. I couldn't get up."

Specific Open-Ended Question/Statement

Nurse: "Tell me more about the dizziness."
Patient: "I woke up this morning and I couldn't get out of bed. I was so dizzy and then I felt sick to my stomach."

Closed-Ended Directed Question

Nurse: "You have been dizzy and nauseous since you woke up today. Have you vomited?"
Patient: "No, I didn't throw up but I sure felt like I could, so I laid down again. I have never felt like this before."

Menu Question

Nurse: "Do you feel the nausea when you are lying down, when you sit up, or when you start to move?"
Patient: "It starts when I begin to move from lying down to sitting up and gets worse if I try to stand up."

Combination of Different Question Styles

Nurse: "That's a scary feeling. When you feel dizzy, do you feel like you can't get your balance or like the room is spinning?" (W/h question with a menu.)

Patient: "It feels like the room is spinning around me."

Nurse: "As you go from lying to standing, you feel like the room is spinning around you. You feel nauseous but you haven't vomited. Do I have this right?" (Directed closed-ended question to summarize the patient's symptoms.)

Patient: "Yes, that's it."

When questioning a patient, nurses often develop a sense of the patient's ability to convey information. Some patients are shy and need more directed questions to help them respond. Others will ramble or be vague, and then the w/h questions will help target the assessment to specific issues. With experience, nurses develop a sense of different communication styles and learn which questions will provide the most detailed and accurate information.

Time

The pace of modern health care does not often allow for long discussions with patients. Questions tend to be more closed ended, or lists are used to shorten the time needed to acquire information. Many patients, such as elderly individuals, might not be able to understand questions that convey information rapidly. If possible, time should be allotted for careful interviewing. The more accurate the assessment or interview, the easier it is to develop appropriate interventions.

Self-Disclosure

The process of interviewing patients often combines the nurse's professional expertise and personal experiences. Patients may share intimate details about their lives, bodies, and feelings with nurses. Revealing these stories requires a certain level of trust, and patients may want to know their nurses better before sharing their personal information. Sometimes they might ask questions that seem inappropriate or too intimate to share within the bounds of a professional relationship. When discerning whether to share personal information, nurses need to remember that the focus of nurse–patient relationships is always on the patient. However, in long-term relationships, such as in a rehabilitation hospital or an outpatient oncology center, some sharing of personal information by nurses may occur as part of ongoing visits. For example, suppose a patient with metastatic breast cancer comes to the oncology center for weekly trastuzumab infusions. Over the course of a year, the patient and the oncology nurse develop a relationship during the infusions with the sharing of some personal information, such as shared interests in literature. While these might be satisfying moments in a nurse's career, it is important to remember, particularly for newer nurses, that the focus of care is always the patient first (Box 6-8).

As discussed in the *Establishing a Therapeutic Relationship* chapter, self-disclosure may be appropriate after the therapeutic relationship is established and both the patient and the nurse understand their roles and the goals of the relationship. The timing of self-disclosure by nurses should always be sensitive to the individual circumstances and patient personalities. Sometimes the relationship between a nurse and a patient is brief and problem focused. For example, in an urgent care clinic, a young patient asks the nurse if she has ever had abdominal pain similar to what the patient is experiencing. The nurse would appropriately redirect the patient by saying, "Let's stay focused on your needs. Tell me more about this pain in your belly." In contrast, if a patient with diabetes has been working with the same nurse for 3 years and she arrives for a routine checkup in December, asking the nurse about holiday plans might be appropriate. Each situation should be approached individually and sensitively to meet the obligations inherent in the nurse's professional role.

With clinical experience, nurses develop a sense of what is appropriately discussed during short- and long-term patient relationships. Self-disclosure is often a gradual process that occurs in steps over time and requires judgment. There is often a desire on the part of the patient to know more about his or her healthcare provider. When patients ask personal questions, it is often because they want to

---

Box 6-8 Rules on Sharing Personal Information

- Do not answer a question that feels uncomfortable. Refocus the interaction on the patient's needs.
- Do not ask a patient for advice on personal issues.
- Never share information about another patient.

know the person to whom they are disclosing their private information. Disclosure and trust are closely related. When patients trust their nurses, they will more readily and honestly talk about their issues. Sharing of more personal details, such as ages of children or favorite foods, might be appropriate in longer, more established relationships. Asking a patient for a recipe might be appropriate, but asking for advice on personal issues is probably never appropriate. The focus should always remain on the patient's needs.

Some of the most satisfying moments in nursing occur during long-term relationships with patients. The sharing of mutual experiences as human beings is meaningful, but the ability to differentiate between appropriate sharing and inappropriate personal questions develops with experience. When newer nurses are unsure about how to answer personal questions from patients, an experienced nurse or colleague may provide advice about the situation. It is best not to share personal information with patients if it feels uncomfortable. Setting boundaries about what is appropriate to discuss as well as the nurse's comfort level with disclosing personal information will help with professional role development and, additionally, focus care on the patient's needs.

Summary

Interviewing skills are part science and part art. To newer nurses trying to evaluate a patient's status, the types of questions that might potentially be asked may seem endless. However, with clinical experience, nurses develop a focused approach to obtaining reliable and useful information from patients. Using a variety of questions and responses, nurses can streamline conversations so that important facts are obtained efficiently and sensitively. Acknowledging the presence and intensity of emotional undertones in patient statements will help patients feel understood and enhance the development of therapeutic relationships.

Case Study Resolution

Mrs. S.'s symptoms—nausea, chest pain, and weeping—could be due to any number of problems, ranging from depression to myocardial infarction. In this case, she had actually experienced a myocardial infarction. The nurse's further questioning allowed for a more accurate description of the symptoms. Mrs. S. had an uneventful recovery from her myocardial infarction, and she was referred to social services for counseling.

EXERCISES

1. Read the following interview between a nurse and a patient. Label each statement by the nurse with the type of response or question used: closed-ended question, open-ended question, menu question, interchangeable response, additive response, ignoring, or minimizing. Note: Some statements or questions may fit into more than one category.

   1. *Patient:* "I can't quit smoking!"
     Nurse: "Of course you can."

   2. *Patient:* "No, you don't understand. I have tried everything, but when I am around my family smoking, I just can't help myself."
     Nurse: "It's hard to quit when your family smokes."

   3. *Patient:* "I just keep trying new things but nothing works."
     Nurse: "You sound frustrated."

   4. *Patient:* "I am."
     Nurse: "Which methods have you tried to quit smoking?"

   5. *Patient:* "I tried the patch and the gum and even went cold turkey."
     Nurse: "Did the patch work for you?"

   6. *Patient:* "No."
     Nurse: "Would you like to join our quit smoking group or try the nicotine gum again?"

   7. *Patient:* "I guess I need both to quit. Do you think it will work?"
     Nurse: "Let's check your blood pressure."

   8. *Patient:* "What other things can I try?"
     Nurse: "Would you like to try the patch again, a newer medicine called varenicline, or an antidepressant called bupropion?"

ANSWERS

   1. Minimizing

   2. Interchangeable response

   3. Additive response

4. Open-ended question

5. Closed-ended question

6. Menu question

7. Ignoring

8. Menu question

2. Active listening is a skill that can be developed. Break into groups of two. One person will be the "storyteller," and the other will be the "listener." The "storyteller" shares a significant life experience with the "listener" in 5 minutes or less. Then the "listener" summarizes the "storyteller's" life experience. The "storyteller" then either validates the story or clarifies it.

- Did the "listener" accurately relay the facts of the story? Which information was missing or heard incorrectly?
- Did the "listener" use attentive body language? (Were his or her arms crossed? Did he or she maintain good eye contact?)
- Did the "listener" remember the feelings or emotions that were part of the story?
- Why was this experience significant to the "storyteller"?

Websites

American Academy on Communication in Healthcare, Demonstration module, "Build the Relationship":

http://webcampus.drexelmed.edu/doccom/user/static/m_06_demo/default_FrameSet.htm

American Psychiatric Nurses Association:

http://www.apna.org/i4a/pages/index.cfm?pageid=3334#sthash.SFYX7DvE.dpbs

Evidence-Based Article

Gallagher, R., Trotter, R., & Donoghue, J. (2010). Preprocedural concerns and anxiety assessment in patients undergoing coronary angiography and percutaneous coronary interventions. *European Journal of Cardiovascular Nursing, 9*, 38–44.

Patients may experience anxiety before coronary procedures that may have a negative consequence. In this study described in this article, 159 patients were surveyed using two measures of anxiety: the Spielberger State Anxiety Inventory and the Faces Anxiety Scale. The patient levels of anxiety were found to be low to moderate, with the biggest concern being the outcome of the procedure. Patients taking medicine for anxiety, those with major concerns about the outcome, and those experiencing angina had higher anxiety scores. The authors recommend routine assessment of anxiety in these patients with appropriate management.

References

Arnold, E. C., & Boggs, K. U. (2011). *Interpersonal relationships: Professional communication skills for nurses* (6th ed.). St. Louis, MO: Elsevier Saunders.

Fortin, A. H., Dwamena, F. C., Framkel, R. M., & Smith, R. C. (2012). 5-step patient-centered interviewing. In *Smith's patient-centered interviewing: An evidence-based method* (p. 30). New York: McGraw-Hill.

Greene, J. O., & Burleson, B. R. (2003). Communication in healthcare contexts. In *Handbook of communication and social interaction skills* (pp. 921–923). Mahwah NJ: Lawrence Erlbaum Associates.

Riley, J. B. (2012). Asking questions. In *Communication in nursing* (7th ed., p. 143). St. Louis, MO: Elsevier Mosby.

Sheldon, L. K., Barrett, R., & Ellington, L. (2006). Difficult communication in nursing. *Journal of Nursing Scholarship, 38*(2), 141–147.

CHAPTER SEVEN

Nonverbal Communication: Cues and Body Language

Lisa Kennedy Sheldon

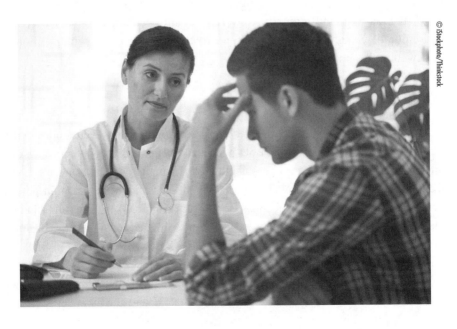

■ **CASE STUDY**

Mr. O., a 60-year-old man with a long history of schizophrenia, has walked into the local community health center complaining of a cough. The nurse, John, has known Mr. O. for 3 years and finds it difficult to communicate with him. In the past, Mr. O. has had unexpected angry outbursts or begun to stare at the floor and not respond to questions, making it difficult to assess his condition. When he is told that Mr. O. is in exam room 3, John reluctantly approaches the room and stands in the doorway. Mr. O. is sitting in the exam room chair, looking at the floor. John leans against the door, crosses his arms around the chart, and says to Mr. O., "How can I help you today?"

Introduction

Nonverbal communication is often described as the process of relaying or receiving information without sounds. It may account for more than half of all communication. In health care, attention to nonverbal cues may be used to interpret the verbal communication. These unspoken cues may add to, undo, or contradict the verbal communication (Giger & Davidhizar, 2008). Nonverbal cues may include both body language, such as touch or posture, and verbal qualities, such as tone and volume. Nonverbal communication may vary by person and cultural background. The types and roles of nonverbal communication are reviewed in this chapter.

Body Language

Body posture, arm position, hand gestures, eye contact, and even smiles can all convey messages without words. Both nurses and patients use body language, often unconsciously, to transmit messages about their willingness to communicate or their fears and concerns (Arnold & Boggs, 2011). Patients might adapt certain postures that indicate vulnerability or openness to conversation. Nurses, too, might indicate their interest through their posture and gestures. In the case study at the beginning of the chapter, John is showing cautiousness or a lack of true interest in Mr. O. by staying in the door instead of coming into the room and by clasping his arms around the chart. In nursing, body language plays an important role in building rapport with patients, and certain body postures may not facilitate disclosure by patients.

Evaluating body language is a part of active listening and provides relevant data about the patient that are useful in assessment, diagnosis, treatment, education, and counseling (Fortin, Dwamena, Framkel, & Smith, 2012). In this section, several types of body language are reviewed:

- Facial expressions and eye contact
- Hand and arm gestures
- Posture
- Body space
- Touch

Facial Expressions and Eye Contact

The face can convey surprise, interest, anger, sadness, joy, or fear. Facial expressions may be consistent with the actual verbal message, or, if not, they may require reinterpretation of the spoken words. When the facial expression and the verbal message are the same, there is congruence between the words and the meaning (Greene & Burleson, 2003). In such a case, the nonverbal cues from facial expressions serve to reinforce the spoken words. The face can also convey strong emotions, such as anger and surprise, or the face may be quiet or masklike. A smile usually conveys warmth and openness when used in the appropriate circumstances; conversely, a smile in the wrong situation may be very disconcerting. Whereas some facial expressions are easier to read, such as downcast eyes and tears, others can be more ambiguous. Lack of appropriate facial expression should be noted during the nursing assessment because some diseases such as Parkinson's disease and some psychiatric disorders can cause a flattening of affect and minimize facial expressions.

Confirmation with the patient is an important component of assessing nonverbal communication because of the individual variation in expressions. Statements such as "You look worried to me" or "You seem uncomfortable" may be used to validate the nurse's assessment of the patient's thoughts and feelings. Statements of appraisal also denote a willingness to try to understand the patient's concerns and a sincere interest in the patient.

There is significant cultural variation in facial expressions, especially eye contact. What may be acceptable in one culture may be considered offensive in another. For example, people from some cultural backgrounds may interpret the raising of the eyebrows or a direct gaze as hostile or insulting. Others, such as dominant-culture Americans, may view direct eye contact as conveying interest, openness, or trustworthiness. Sometimes prolonged eye contact, especially in conjunction with physical touch, is viewed as a sign of intimacy. A downward glance might be a sign of respect, as seen in people who identify themselves as Asian/ Pacific Islanders. It is important to view each patient both as an individual and as a product of his or her cultural background when determining the appropriate methods of nonverbal communication.

Hand and Arm Gestures

Gestures with the hands and arms may convey information about both the message and the messenger. Open hands and arms may demonstrate openness and honesty when communicating with others. Folded arms and closed hands or laced fingers might indicate a reticence to talk or to divulge personal information. Crossed arms might also indicate a sense of vulnerability and a need for self-protection. Evaluating hand and arm gestures may provide clues about how the patient is feeling and what his or her preferred communication style is. Also, nurses may convey messages to their patients with their gestures, such as in the case study at the beginning of the chapter. Using open body language may indicate to patients that nurses are willing to engage with them and desire to understand their concerns.

Body Posture

Body posture may indicate how receptive one person feels toward another. Being seated or leaning toward another person (as when a nurse actively listens to a patient) demonstrates an interest in what that individual is saying. Rigid posture, in contrast, might convey a reluctance to engage in meaningful conversation. Crossed legs could be interpreted as self-protection, or they could be a position of comfort if all other nonverbal and verbal communication indicates openness. Tapping feet might indicate nervousness or impatience and could be an indicator of blocked communication. The nurse needs to be aware of the patient's body posture as well as his or her own when communicating with patients.

Body Space

Body space varies with the type of relationship between people and cultural background. Social distance is usually considered to be approximately 3 to 4 feet between people (Table 7-1); such distance is used in conversations between

Table 7-1 Social Spaces

Space	Distance	Context
Intimate	Physical contact to 18 inches away	Reserved for close, personal relationships, but nurses often enter this space during routine care
Personal	18 inches to 4 feet	Used in friendships, but occurs often when delivering nursing care
Social	4 to 12 feet	Used in everyday life and business
Public	Greater than 12 feet	Used during lectures and speeches

acquaintances and in business relationships. It is also used by nurses during interactions with patients. Often, nursing care requires nurses to come closer to patients to perform physical care or medical interventions. If time allows, it is best for nurses to ask patients for permission to come closer during the first encounters or, at the minimum, inform them of what is about to happen. This notice allows patients to prepare for a change in acceptable spaces and sets the tone for relationships where patients are in control of their surroundings and participate in decisions regarding their care.

Be aware that different circumstances may change the amount of space between the nurse and the patient. An anxious patient or a patient with psychiatric issues might need more space to feel comfortable. Patients who are in pain or undergoing a procedure might need the nurse to be closer or to use touch to reassure them. Holding a hand or giving a gentle touch on the arm, if appropriate, might make the patient more at ease during stressful times. Each patient is unique, with different body space requirements. Each situation requires assessment and adjustment to make the patient feel safe and comfortable.

Cultural differences might also change the body space requirements. Americans, Britons, and Canadians need greater personal space than Hispanic Americans, Africans, and Arabs. For example, North American, Indian, African American, Asian, and Pakistani cultures may require greater personal space than Hispanics, southern Europeans, and Arabs (Richmond, McCroskey, & Payne, 1987).

Touch

Touch can communicate many messages (Box 7-1). The use of touch is the universal language of caring. It can transcend age or language differences. Reaching out physically shows concern for another human being. Touch is a powerful tool.

Box 7-1	Uses of Touch

- Refocus patients who are rambling or self-absorbed
- Reduce anxiety in stressful situations
- Convey interest in the patient's experience
- Create human connections
- Express caring
- Provide physical care

Nurses use touch in a variety of ways—some comforting, others as part of necessary physical care and interventions. The use of touch can reassure, calm, and support patients. For example, holding the hand of a woman in labor indicates support and caring during intense contractions. Nurses use touch to directly care for their patients, such as during bathing or changing positions. However, touch may also be uncomfortable, such as during the insertion of an intravenous catheter. A firm touch may be interpreted as controlling or hostile. Prior to any invasive or painful form of touch, a trusting relationship needs to be established.

Touch can be misconstrued as sexual by some patients. Caution should be used with patients during physical care such as perineal cleaning, and the meaning of the touch should be explained to avoid misunderstandings. As a general rule, touching above the elbow, when not part of physical care, can be confusing to some patients. Careful assessment of the patients' need for space and their reaction to touch is necessary to prevent awkwardness and embarrassment.

Summary

Nonverbal communication and body language can relay important information during interactions. Patients often convey their feelings and concerns without words, requiring the nurse to carefully assess both what is said and what remains unspoken. Evaluating body language is a part of active listening and provides information about patients that is useful in assessment, diagnosis, treatment, education, and counseling. Nurses also convey messages to patients with their body posture, which may either facilitate or block patient communication. Understanding the role of nonverbal communication is an important part of nursing assessment and intervention.

Touch, when used appropriately, may communicate caring, reduce anxiety, and make connections between nurses and patients.

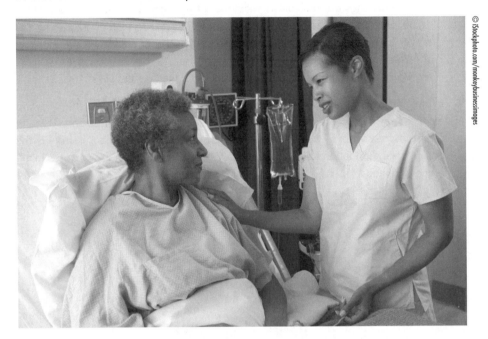

Case Study Resolution

The nurse's words were appropriate, but everything else conveyed a reluctance to engage with Mr. O. The crossed arms and position in the doorway did not demonstrate a willingness to become involved in Mr. O.'s care. All patients, but particularly those who have difficulty relating to others, such as individuals with schizophrenia, need to sense attention and concern on the part of the nurse. Entering the room with an open posture would have been a better way to begin the encounter with Mr. O.

EXERCISES

1. Break into groups of three, with each group having a video camera, if possible. One student can be the "nurse," one can be the "patient," and one can be the "videographer." In 5 minutes, role-play and videotape the following scenario. Have the "nurse" interview the "patient" about healthy behaviors (e.g., smoking, alcohol consumption, nutrition, sleep, checkups). Then watch the videotape as a group, paying attention to the nonverbal behaviors of the "nurse" and "patient."

- Which behaviors indicate a willingness to communicate on the part of the nurse?
- Which behaviors indicate a willingness to communicate on the part of the patient?
- Which postures convey a reluctance to participate for each?
- Which nonverbal postures did the "nurse" use?
- Which types of nonverbal communication did the "patient" use?

2. Expressing feelings without words can be a challenge. Write each of the following emotions on a separate slip of paper and distribute one to each person. Then, in 1 minute or less, have each person act out the emotion on the paper in front of the group. Face, hands, and body can be used, but not any sounds or words (as in the game Charades).

- Happiness
- Anger
- Sadness
- Frustration
- Shock
- Uncertainty
- Confidence
- Disinterest
- Reluctance
- Acceptance
- Disapproval

QUESTIONS

- Which emotions were most difficult to portray with nonverbal cues?
- Could some nonverbal cues have more than one interpretation?
- Which emotions were easy to "read"?
- How would cultural diversity change the meaning of some nonverbal communication? How will you approach patients in your care?

Websites

American Academy on Communication in Healthcare:
https://aachonline.site-ym.com/default.asp?

Evidence-Based Article

O'Lynn, C., & Krautscheid, L. (2011). How should I touch? A qualitative study of attitudes on intimate touch in nursing care. *American Journal of Nursing, 111*(3), 24–31.

In this study, the researchers interviewed 24 people about their preferences for touching by nurses. They explored *intimate touch*—that is, touching of those private body parts that may cause the patient embarrassment. In particular, they explored participants' preferences for touch by male nurses. The themes from the interviews included "Communicate with me," "Give me choices," Ask me about gender," and "Touch me professionally." Participants varied in their preferences for gender. They wanted to be touched firmly but not roughly, and wanted to nurses to ensure their privacy.

References

Arnold, E. C., & Boggs, K. U. (2011). *Interpersonal relationships: Professional communication skills for nurses* (6th ed.). St. Louis, MO: Elsevier Saunders.

Fortin, A. H., Dwamena, F. C., Framkel, R. M., & Smith, R .C. (2012). 5-step patient-centered interviewing. In *Smith's patient-centered interviewing: An evidence-based method* (p. 30). New York: McGraw-Hill.

Giger, J., & Davidhizar, R.. (2008). Nonverbal communication. In J. Giger & R. Davidhizar (Eds.), *Transcultural nursing: Assessment and intervention* (5th ed., pp. 29–33). New York: Mosby.

Greene, J. O., & Burleson, B. R. (2003). Nonverbal communication skills and nonverbal messages. In *Handbook of communication and social interaction skills* (pp. 179–219). Mahwah, NJ: Lawrence Erlbaum Associates.

Richmond, V., McCroskey, J., & Payne, S. (1987). *Nonverbal behavior in interpersonal relations*. Englewood Cliffs, NJ: Prentice Hall.

CHAPTER EIGHT

Humor

Lisa Kennedy Sheldon
Janice B. Foust

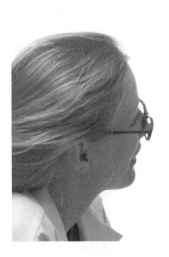
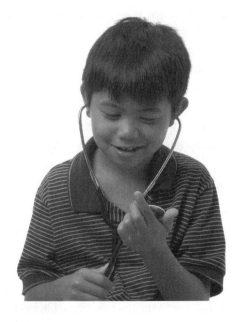

■ **CASE STUDY**

J.J., a 7-year-old boy, is hospitalized for a broken femur, requiring placement of pins and traction. J.J. rings the call bell, and the nurse responds to him through the intercom in the wall speaker behind his bed. J.J. says, "What do you want, Wall?" This begins a regular joke between J.J. and the nurse. The nurse would call herself "Mrs. Wall," and J.J. found this very amusing.

Introduction

One of the most delightful aspects of human interaction is the use of humor. It can lift the spirits, free people from their everyday routines, and create human connections. Humor can put people at ease, celebrate shared victories, relieve tension, reveal shared foibles, and even promote learning. It is also an important communication tool in the nurse–patient relationship. When used appropriately and judiciously, humor can provide new perspectives on the challenges of life and create bonds between people. What is amusing may be individual, but the ability to laugh is shared by all human beings.

For example, an oncology nurse in the outpatient office is trying to assess Mr. R.'s bowel function, but the patient in a semi-private room next to Mr. R. is quite close in proximity. When the nurse lowers her voice to discuss stool softeners, the adjacent patient yells out from behind the curtain, "Oh, I used that stuff and I've been regular ever since." The two patients begin a lively discussion about different stool softeners. The humor of the situation is not lost on any of them, and a good laugh is shared by all.

There are several different types of humor, however, and not all are appropriate in the nurse–patient relationship. Types of humor include positive humor, negative humor, and black humor (Riley, 2012, pp. 163–173).

Positive Humor

Positive humor is the type that builds relationships and releases tension. It is constructive and joyful, creative and gentle. For example, a nurse hands a woman a gown and tells her to leave it open in the back, and then hands her a second gown and tells her it's the robe, so she can have an elegant, matching set. This is positive humor, based on the well-known ridiculousness of hospital gowns. It breaks the tension of disrobing and (the nurse hopes) brings a smile to the patient.

Nurses can use positive humor to share joy and humility. The highest form of humor is the ability to laugh at oneself. It shows perspective and reassures patients that we all have imperfections. Humor based on humility allows us to share our humanness with others. In another scenario, an inpatient is complaining about the hospital food on his tray, when the dietician says, "What do you want for $500 a day?"

Negative Humor

Negative humor, unlike positive humor, is not helpful. It makes people feel uncomfortable, demeaned, or defensive. It usually involves sarcasm or put-downs, or has stereotype, racist, ageist, or sexist undertones that might be offensive or hurtful. While it could temporarily relieve tension, negative humor is unprofessional and disrespectful and should not be used during any nurse–patient interactions.

Black Humor

The use of "black humor" among hospital staff may provide relief during tense situations. Hospital staff often deals with intense and dramatic situations that involve the whole spectrum of health and illness, from spilled bodily excrement to nudity and death. Black humor provides a psychological escape from the harsh realities and may even strengthen staff relationships. These shared experiences can provide "comic relief" from some of the absurd and frightening realities of working in health care.

One note: Black humor should never be shared with the patients and should be used cautiously among staff. The nurse needs to be prepared for patients who may use this type of humor to relieve tension or anxiety about potentially life-threatening situations. Such a nurse can use these comments to open up discussion and provide reassurance, clarify misunderstandings, and provide support. However, even if the patient seems comfortable with black humor, it is important that the nurse try not to encourage it.

Appropriate Use of Humor

When is it appropriate to use humor as an intervention in health care? As with much of life, timing and context are everything. Pertinent factors include how long the nurse has known the patient, the patient's age, the patient's personality (e.g., extrovert versus introvert), and the acuity of the clinical situation. Humor may be culturally different, so understanding the patient's cultural background is important to avoid offending patients (Giger & Davidhizar, 2008). Humor in healthcare settings is intended to be therapeutic and is not disparaging, sarcastic, or cynical (Box 8-1). Patients should never be the focus of the humor. A coworker who uses humor effectively with patients may be an inspiration and a teacher.

It is important to understand the patient's perspective when deciding when to use humor (Greene & Burleson, 2003). Nurses are very familiar with their clinical settings and routine, but those elements may be puzzling or uncomfortable for patients. However, if nurses put themselves in a patient's situation, they may see situations that can be tactfully handled with humor. For example, one may use humor to acknowledge the awkwardness of hospital gowns or routine procedures (e.g., pulse oximetry). Trying a simple joke, such as in the gown scenario, helps the nurse assess the patient's response to levity and his or her clinical situation. Some patients and families, particularly during emergency or critical situations, will understandably feel that their care is not being taken seriously if the nurse tells a joke at the wrong time. Nurses should be alert to evaluating the patient's response to humor. If the patient appears offended or did not respond to the humor, the nurse should apologize and reassure the patient that it was an attempt to be helpful or to put him or her at ease.

Patients set the tone of the conversation, and the nurse needs to respond accordingly. Patients might joke about their disease by calling it a name, especially if they have been living with it for a while. For example, a female patient with chronic lymphocytic leukemia might say, "Luke is back," when her white blood cell count starts rising, indicating the need for more chemotherapy.

Nurses should have the ability to laugh at themselves and with their patients. Be open to different forms of interaction with patients, including humor, to develop a personal style of communication with patients that is unique, effective, and rewarding.

Box 8-1 Uses of Humor

- Begin interaction
- Put the patient at ease
- Convey joy
- Lighten the atmosphere and relieve tension
- Reveal our weaknesses and humanity
- Acknowledge the absurdities of life and/or situations

Summary

Humor may be a useful tool when communicating with patients. It needs to be used judiciously and based on the nurses' assessment of the patient's needs and the context of the situation, however (Table 8-1). Humor is used on an individual basis, and nurses should be aware of some the nuances associated with using humor with patients and also why patients may be joking with them. When used

Table 8-1 Strategies for Using Humor

Strategy	Example
Start with gentle humor.	When a patient tries to talk while you are taking a blood pressure, the nurse would lift the diaphragm up like a microphone and say, "What was that?"
Try to put the patient at ease during tense situations.	When the nurse has difficulty finding a good site for an intravenous catheter, she says, "Can I give you one of my veins?"
Incorporate humor in teaching.	A nurse struggling to draw a heart to explain valve surgery to a patient says, "Wait until we get to kidneys. I am good at drawing them!"
Make a book of jokes and cartoons to share with patients.	A cartoon shows a woman coming in to the urgent care center. The nurse asks, "What brought you in today?" She looks at her daughter and says "My own personal ambulance."
Use puppets, props, toys, and even bubbles with children (or adults!).	Keep games, such as cards, electronic chess, or checkers, and funny videos to help patients pass the time enjoyably.
Encourage a positive attitude in both patients and staff.	Use group projects such as decorating the department for holidays or create special days like "wear-purple Fridays."
Employ humor with one another.	The staff that laughs together is more productive, and job satisfaction and retention are higher.
Keep jokes simple and playful with children.	"What happens when ducks fly upside down? They quack up!"

effectively, humor may dissipate anxiety and provide some relief to the often-stressful events associated with a change in health.

Case Study Resolution

J.J. remained in traction for 2 weeks, requiring another surgery for internal fixation of his fracture. His relationship with "Mrs. Wall" became an important part of his trust in the nurses. He knew if he talked to the "Wall," then he would receive what he needed, whether it was to relieve his pain or help him go to the bathroom. Sometimes, J.J. just needed to know that the nurse was nearby and hearing her voice was reassuring to him.

EXERCISES

As a group, share some stories about humor as a form of communication:

1. Share some situations where humor was useful and helpful to a patient. What made the use of humor appropriate in these stories? What was the patient's response to the joke or humorous situation?

2. Discuss instances when humor was not appropriate or caused patients distress. Why didn't humor work in each instance? When should a nurse not use a joke with a patient?

3. Talk about "black humor" and how you have seen it used by healthcare professions in the work setting. How do you feel about it? What are the appropriate times to use this form of humor? How does the staff react to black or "gallows" humor?

Evidence-Based Article

Tse, M. M. Y., Lo, A. P. K., Cheng, T. L. Y., Chan, E. K. K., Chan, A. H. Y., & Chung, H. S. W. (2010). Humor therapy: Relieving chronic pain and enhancing happiness for older adults. *Journal of Aging Research.* doi: 10.4061/2010/343574

Older patients in a nursing home were invited to participate in an 8-week humor therapy program. Seventy patients participated in this quasi-experimental study ($n = 36$ experimental group and 34 control group). The participants in the experimental group created a portfolio, "My Happy Folder," filled with jokes, photos, and videos. They also participated in groups where they learned about incorporating humor in their lives. Patients in the experimental group had lower pain scores and higher scores on measures of happiness and life satisfaction and lower scores on loneliness at week 8 of the intervention when compared with the control group. The researchers recommend the use of "My Happy Folder" to help patients manage symptoms such as pain and to allow humor to play a greater role in increasing their enjoyment of life.

References

Giger, J., & Davidhizar, R. (Eds.). (2008). Humor in communication. In *Transcultural nursing: Assessment and intervention* (5th ed., p. 33). New York: Mosby.

Greene, J. O., & Burleson, B. R. (2003). Comprehension processes underlying humor elicitation. In *Handbook of communication and social interaction skills* (pp. 300–302). Mahwah, NJ: Lawrence Erlbaum Associates.

Riley, J. B. (2012). Humor. In *Communication in nursing* (7th ed., pp. 163–173). St. Louis, MO: Elsevier Mosby.

Specific Communication

CHAPTER NINE

Improving Quality of Care and Safety During Transitions in Care

Janice B. Foust

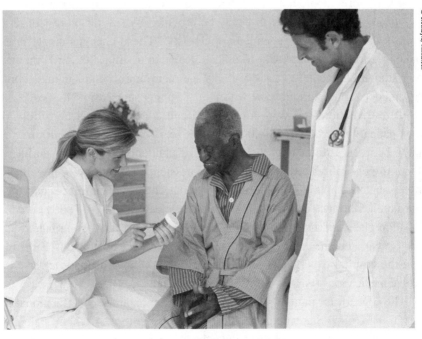

■ CASE STUDY

Mrs. Z. is an 81-year-old woman who was diagnosed with heart failure a year ago. She was admitted to the hospital with complaints of a weight gain of 4 pounds in 1 week, paroxysmal nocturnal dyspnea, and fatigue. Mrs. Z. says she takes her medications but did not take her diuretic for the past 2 days. She "watches" her salt intake. She has bilateral pedal edema and bilateral crackles in one-fourth of her lung fields. Mrs. Z. lives in a 2 story townhouse. Her husband died 2 years ago, and she does not have any children.

Introduction

Patients receive care in very different clinical settings depending on the acuity of patient care needs (e.g., emergency units, hospitals, skilled nursing facilities, outpatient clinic offices). A fragmented healthcare system contributes to costly, poor patient outcomes such as adverse events after patients leave the hospital or lead to unnecessary hospital readmissions. Care transitions are more complicated today than they were years ago for several reasons. Specifically, the U.S. population is aging and more people are living with chronic conditions, requiring increasingly complicated treatment plans that may be provided by several professionals (e.g., primary care providers, specialists, therapists). These changes create practical challenges for interdisciplinary healthcare teams in multiple settings, who need to work smoothly together to assist patients and their families in planning, coordinating, and delivering complex care within increasingly shorter time frames.

Care transitions are very complicated and common. Such transitions occur when patients are transferred within a setting (e.g., intensive care units and general units), between settings (e.g., hospital and rehabilitation centers), or during handoffs of responsibility between healthcare professionals. Another very important (and often simultaneous) transition occurs when the healthcare team teaches patients (and their families) to take care of themselves as they leave a setting. Poorly coordinated transition plans and inadequate communication of those plans contribute to costly, poor patient outcomes. For example, nearly 1 in 5 patients who is discharged home from the hospital experiences an adverse event, and 66% of these adverse events involve medications (Forster, Murff, Peterson, Gandhi, & Bates, 2003).

The concern for patient safety and quality has inspired several national initiatives in the United States (e.g., medication reconciliation). A major quality initiative in the United States seeks to reduce the number of patients who are readmitted within 30 days of hospital discharge (Centers for Medicare and Medicaid, 2012); achieving this goal will require better care coordination. Communication is an essential component of effective care transitions. In addition, healthcare teams must anticipate problems and be proactive when planning and preparing patients (and their families) to leave a setting. This chapter focuses on three communication-related interventions to improve care transitions for those patients who are most likely to experience problems: (1) targeted assessment of common transition-related problems, (2) patient and family education, and (3) communication among professionals as they relate to posthospital transitions.

Models to Improve Care Transitions

Studies of transitional care and redesigned hospital discharge processes indicate that it is possible to improve patient outcomes and reduce costs of care by targeting care transitions. Transitional care has been "defined as a set of actions designed to ensure the coordination and continuity of healthcare as patients transfer between different locations or different levels of care within the same location" and includes patient and family education (Coleman & Boult, 2003, p. 556).

Hospital readmissions are reduced when either an advanced practice nurse or transitions coach provides transitional care for patients who are discharged home from the hospital (Coleman, Parry, Chalmers, & Min, 2006; Naylor et al., 1999; Naylor et al., 2004). A *transitions coach* empowers patients and their families to take a more active role in posthospital transitions based on the four pillars of care—that is, medication management, personal health record, red flags, and follow-up care (Coleman et al., 2006). Another model, the transitional care model, features a *transitional care nurse* who leads a multidisciplinary approach to provide comprehensive in-hospital discharge planning and home follow-up for high-risk, chronically ill older adults that emphasizes preventing complications and improving patient outcomes (Transitional Care Model, 2008–2009). Both of these transitional care models emphasize coordination and continuity of care among healthcare professionals who work closely with patients and their families to improve patient outcomes.

Other researchers have redesigned hospital discharge processes to improve posthospital transitions (Balaban, Weissman, Samuel, & Woodhandler, 2008; Jack et al., 2009). To do so, they standardized aspects of discharge processes such as discharge instructions, medication reconciliation, and posthospital appointments with primary care providers and/or telephone follow-up by a nurse or pharmacist. These actions have been shown to reduce hospital utilization and improve patients' attendance at posthospital appointments.

All of these models of care highlight the benefits of improved care coordination, better patient education prior to discharge, and posthospital follow-up strategies aimed at chronically ill patients. Nurses play a vital role in improving the quality and safety of care transitions.

Targeted Assessment of Common Transition-Related Problems

Nurses are in an ideal position to identify the problems whose resolution is most likely to improve care transitions. In the course of their clinical interactions with patients and families, nurses are likely to learn how patients have been managing their health, uncover misunderstandings, or discover limited resources that can be critical sources of care transition problems. Screening tools directed toward discharge planning are available and tremendously helpful to begin the care transition process and identify those individuals who would benefit from services after hospital discharge (Bixby & Naylor, 2009; Holland, Harris, Leibson, Pankratz, & Kirchbaum, 2006). Whether guided by a discharge screening tool or standardized admission assessment, nurses need to ask relevant questions to identify issues that may delay hospital discharge or contribute to hospital readmission.

It is essential to identify problems early enough in the hospital admission to allow the healthcare team to collaboratively plan and coordinate necessary interventions with the healthcare providers, patients, and their families. Healthcare professionals often (and understandably) focus their clinical assessments on immediate problems and risk factors of the acute care situation at hand. As a result, some of the most critical transition-related questions are too rarely asked or, when asked, are not allocated sufficient time for the healthcare team to develop an effective plan (Table 9-1). In essence, effective care transitions rely on proactive and timely assessments that give the healthcare team enough time to address the patient's unique needs and collaboratively develop and communicate the plan with the patient, family, and posthospital healthcare professionals.

Problems can arise from many different sources during care transitions. It can be difficult for healthcare professionals to anticipate problems when they are not familiar

Table 9-1 Too Rarely Asked Questions (TRAQ): Assessments and Interdisciplinary Implications

Topic	Patient Assessment	Interdisciplinary Care Transition Implications
Signs and symptoms	• Which signs or symptoms were experienced? • How long had these signs or symptoms occurred?	Identifies the most obvious and bothersome signs or symptoms to be addressed. Specifically, enables providers to develop plans for early sign/symptom recognition with associated action plans.
	• Which actions were taken to alleviate these signs or symptoms?	Determine effective interventions—when used.
	• What, if anything, helped?	Discharge instructions should address what patients should expect to experience and do for themselves, once they are home.
Self-management strategies	• Describe a typical day and how you manage your health (e.g., activity, nutrition, medications).	Develop individualized discharge instructions to fit the patient's routines and preferences.
	• What are sources of support and challenges? What are sources of frustration or barriers?	Address sources of problems such as financial or transportation limitations with community referrals.
Medication management	• Which medications were taken before admission? Compared to discharge?	Interdisciplinary medication reconciliation processes and problem solving. Patient and family education that highlights issues such as medication: – Names (both brand and generic) – Any changes (e.g., new medications, increased or decreased doses or frequencies) – Schedule – Side effects – Follow-up actions or needed monitoring On the day of discharge, identify what needs to be taken once at home (because the patient likely received medications that day in the hospital). Encourage the patient to maintain a current medication list and bring it to all healthcare appointments.
	• What is the medication insurance plan? • Which pharmacy does the patient use?	Insurance – Formulary issues (i.e., generic, brand) – May need preauthorization for certain medications

(continued)

Table 9-1 Too Rarely Asked Questions (TRAQ): Assessments and Interdisciplinary Implications (*continued*)

Topic	Patient Assessment	Interdisciplinary Care Transition Implications
		Prescriptions: – May need to fax prescriptionsMay need two sets of prescriptions (local pharmacy and mail order) – May need caregiver to pick up medications before discharge – Does the local pharmacy have the medication available (if unusual or costly)?
Home environment	Describe the physical layout of the home setting: – Stairs? Elevator? – Access to bathtub, shower? – Screen for risks (e.g. falls)	Develop plan activities to accommodate the patient's environment. May need consultations for home modifications. Address safety issues.
Family caregiver involvement	Who does patient rely on? Where do caregivers live (i.e., nearby)? What do caregivers do to help?	Identify the support network. As the patient indicates, provide for early and continuous involvement of the appropriate caregiver in teaching and planning.
Transportation	Available transportation for appointments? Shopping?	May need referral for community support or resources.
Posthospital follow-up	Who is the primary care provider? Specialists? Home healthcare clinicians?	Arrange posthospital medical appointments. Communicate the discharge plan and follow-up actions (i.e., pending issues) to all appropriate healthcare professionals.

with patients' unique home environments or problems they typically face once they are home. Table 9-1 identifies some practical assessment topics and their associated implications for care transitions. Specifically, nurses and the healthcare team should assess the following areas: (1) signs and symptoms management, (2) self-management strategies, (3) medication management, (4) the home environment, (5) family caregiver involvement, (6) transportation, and (7) posthospital follow-up.

The patient's ability to resume self-management after being discharged from the hospital is one of the most complicated—and important—aspects of effective care transitions. Nurses have ample opportunities to address these issues as they work with patients and families at the bedside. Nurses observe patients' responses to their illness, their understanding of the treatment plan and health condition, their knowledge of medications and their use, and other self-management activities. Nurses can ask patients which strategies they use at home, which problems they anticipate encountering in the posthospital environment, and when and who they call if there is a problem. Early and targeted assessments will reveal critical information and help to design individualized and effective plans, thereby improving care transitions and patient outcomes. Patients need to be involved in designing a treatment plan that fits their abilities, resources (e.g., financial, community, social support), home environments, and lifestyles.

Patient and Family Education

In the United States, The Joint Commission requires hospital professionals to provide patients and their families with the necessary instructions to promote continuity of care (Joint Commission, 2010). The day of discharge is a very busy time for both healthcare professionals and patients. Patients are often eager to go home, yet they may not feel well and might have difficulty learning or absorbing all the discharge information they are being given both verbally and as written instructions. In addition, patients or family members may not think of questions until they are at home and starting to implement the prescribed plan, which explains why posthospital follow-up calls or visits are important components of transitional care models. Patients are frequently given contact information for who to call with identified problems (e.g., fever), but they may not feel comfortable initiating the call. Nurses should help patients and families become more comfortable with contacting professionals when they have questions so the problem can be managed as early as possible, thereby enabling patients to avoid unnecessary visits to the emergency room or readmission to the hospital.

Discharge teaching ideally begins as soon as the patient is admitted to the hospital so that the patient will become familiar with the plan and what to expect after discharge. Nurses need to identify the learning priorities, deliver understandable information at a proper pace, and identify follow-up learning needs and/or referrals, as needed. To improve patient–provider communication, the National Patient Safety Foundation (2013) initiated an Ask Me 3 campaign that focuses on three questions: (1) What is my main problem? (2) What do I need to do? (3) Why is it important for me to do this? This initiative focuses on providing patients with the information they need to know to care for themselves and the reasons why they need to take certain steps.

Unfortunately, family caregivers may not be involved in the discharge from the hospital as much as they would like (Foust, Vuckovic, & Henriquez, 2012; Graham, Ivey, & Neuhauser, 2009). Nurses should ask patients to identify family caregivers (or others) who help them and what they do to assist the patient. With the patient's permission, nurses should reach out to these family caregivers as early as possible in the hospitalization and involve them throughout the discharge planning process.

Often, the hospital discharge treatment plan includes recommendations that affect patients' daily routines and lifestyles. These steps may be difficult to implement all at once. Motivational interviewing is a useful strategy employed by professionals who are working with patients living with chronic conditions as they make important health-related changes in their lives (Rudak, Sandbœk, Lauritzen, & Christensen, 2005). In this collaborative approach, healthcare professionals work with a patient to create a change while respecting that person's values, choices, and autonomy. Motivational interviewing is more likely to be effective as a discharge teaching strategy because it engages the patient in problem solving in ways that may reveal unanticipated or practical barriers (e.g., financial or transportation issues, physical limitations) that can be addressed or for which the plan can be modified.

Effective discharge teaching addresses both immediate and overall treatment plan considerations. The most common hospital discharge instructions include (1) symptom management, and when and who to call if there are problems; (2) medication regimens; (3) diet and activity restrictions; and (4) follow-up care. Medication issues are some of the most immediate (within 24 hours) concerns faced by patients and their families, such as filling prescriptions and knowing the medication doses and schedules. Patients often passively receive medications in the hospital, but they may not know (or remember) what they took in the hospital, which makes it difficult for them to know what they should take once they are at home. Other practical considerations include situations in which patients are given prescriptions to be filled, but the pharmacy may not be open or have the medication available. Several other posthospital medication issues should be addressed to promote safer care as well (Foust, Naylor, Boling, & Capuzzo, 2005).

Another very important and immediate issue for the posthospital patient is signs and symptoms self-management. For example, patients may be expected to monitor for specific signs or symptoms (e.g., incision, temperature) when they first get home. It is important that the patient has the necessary equipment (e.g., a thermometer) and can report the necessary data back to the nurse—and knows when and who to call with questions or concerns. The nurse should emphasize the importance of *early* recognition and intervention (e.g., calling the primary care provider) as means help to prevent unnecessary hospitalizations. and improve patient outcomes.

Communication Among Professionals

Each professional discipline makes substantial contributions to designing an effective care transition that addresses the complex needs of individual patients. Nurses have a central role in raising relevant questions, relaying patient or family concerns, and promoting collaborative problem solving among diverse professionals. Table 9-1 identifies common issues of transition plans that require collaboration and possible referrals to community resources (e.g., home health care, home modifications). Collaboration and coordinating care with others requires a clear focus on patient needs to improve outcomes, significant time, and vigilant efforts to follow up and assure the plan is implemented. As advocates, nurses make substantial contributions to this process when they communicate the patient's needs and consequences of improving care transitions with appropriate professionals.

Use of structured communication tools (e.g., SBAR), which are more often deployed in acute or emergency situations would also help nurses collaborate on discharge plans with other professionals (see Chapter 18 for more information on SBAR). Although care transition problems are usually not urgent, they are critically important to improve patient outcomes and ensure cost-effective care. Unique aspects of care transition collaborations are the focus on the benefits of early action to prevent complications and description of the potential consequences of delayed action or inaction that might be deleterious to the patient. It is essential to make the connections between current interventions and future patient outcomes.

Nurse-to-nurse communication and collaboration facilitate timely and effective care transitions (see Chapter 18 for more detail). Traditional shift reports (i.e., "hand-offs") provide valuable opportunities for nurses to discuss transition plans, share relevant issues and unresolved problems, and provide an update on the status of patient and family education efforts. Such reports enhance continuity of care and make it more efficient for oncoming nurses to build on team efforts without unnecessary duplication. Interagency referrals include nurse-to-nurse communication as a means to improve patient outcomes. Similar to discharge instructions, written referral forms to a new healthcare setting should identify all components of the treatment plan. It is especially helpful for referring nurses to communicate what has proved effective or ineffective in the patient's care so receiving nurses do not have to "relearn" what works or does not work for an individual patient. To promote efficiency and continuity, referring nurses should also communicate relevant information (e.g., recent laboratory data) that will not be immediately available to receiving healthcare teams and the patients and family education efforts.

Case Study Resolution

After conducting a targeted assessment, the nurse learns that Mrs. Z. did not take her diuretic because she ran out of the medication. She cannot get to the pharmacy, and she relies on her nephew to pick up her prescriptions. He was on a business trip and planned to pick up the prescription on the day she was admitted to the hospital. The nurse also learns that Mrs. Z. "hates" to measure her weight and be "reminded of that number." She is on a low-sodium diet and prepares her own meals when she "feels up to it." Mrs. Z. is not familiar with reading nutritional labels, and her niece does the grocery shopping for her every week.

Based on this assessment, the nurse works with the healthcare team to develop a patient education plan that addresses three priorities in Mrs. Z.'s care: (1) preventing gaps in medication refills and understanding of the reasons for taking her medications; (2) procedure and rationale of daily weight, including how it relates to early interventions; and (3) low-sodium diet. Using principles of motivational interviewing, the nurse works with Mrs. Z. to develop how these issues can be managed within her own setting, resources, and lifestyle. Some of the solutions to prevent gaps in medications could be the use of reminders on calendars and including the nephew in the conversations. In addition, the nurse could work with Mrs. Z. to make sure she has a working scale that she can easily read, is comfortable with its location, and understands how daily weight measurements can be fit into her usual morning routines. A key aspect of the conversation with Mrs. Z is to emphasize how this action—and calling her primary care provider with early signs of change—can prevent her from returning to the hospital, an outcome that presumably she wants to avoid. The nurse could also use role-playing or pose different scenarios and work with Mrs. Z. on when she should call her primary care provider and what she should say. Finally, the nurse has identified a problem with nutrition plans and reading labels that could be addressed with a consult to the dietician and use of appropriate patient educational materials.

Websites

Care Transitions Model

In this model, a transitions coach works with patients and their families to manage transitions across settings and address hand-offs between healthcare professionals.

http://www.caretransitions.org/

Motivational Interviewing

This website is a resource for clinicians and others to learn about motivational interviewing (MI). Although it focuses on clients with substances disorders, it also contains general information about MI that provides a good overview of the principles.

http://www.motivationalinterview.org/

National Patient Safety Foundation, Ask Me 3 Program

This program is designed to promote better patient education to improve patient outcomes. It also has resources related to health literacy.

http://www.npsf.org/for-healthcare-professionals/programs/ask-me-3/

Next Steps in Care

This website has valuable resources for professionals and family caregivers to help them prepare and plan care transitions. Information is available in several languages.

http://www.nextstepincare.org/

North Carolina Health Literacy Program

This website has various tools to assess health literacy and teaching aids. It also provides a valuable teaching tool for professionals to help patients and their families living with heart failure, chronic obstructive lung disease, or diabetes.

http://nchealthliteracy.org/index.html

Transitional Care Model

In this model, a transitional care nurse is the primary coordinator of care among the healthcare team and works closely with patients and their families to provide continuity of care across settings.

http://www.transitionalcare.info/index.html

Transitional Care Model: Hospital Discharge Screening Criteria for High-Risk Older Adults

This screening tool may be used to identify older adults who are most vulnerable to poor outcomes during care transitions.

http://consultgerirn.org/uploads/File/trythis/try_this_26.pdf

Evidence-Based Article

Graham, C. L., Ivey, S. L, & Neuhauser, L. (2009). From hospital to home: Assessing transitional care needs of vulnerable seniors. *Gerontologist, 49*(1), 23–33.

This qualitative study describes the experiences of ethnic, cultural, or language diverse informal caregivers for older adults discharged home from the hospital. The researchers address issues of inadequate caregiver training, inadequate information from hospital discharge planners, and reliance on informal supports. In addition, they describe unique needs of caregivers from diverse backgrounds, such as the role of family in providing care and a lack of linguistically appropriate information and services. One of the nursing implications, appropriate to this chapter, is the need to assess informal supports, involve informal caregivers as soon as possible, and provide them with more information and training.

References

Balaban, R. B., Weissman, J. S., Samuel, P. A., & Woodhandler, S. (2008). Redefining and redesigning hospital discharge to enhance patient care: A randomized controlled study. *Journal of General Internal Medicine, 23*(8), 1228–1233.

Bixby, M. B., & Naylor, M. D. (2009). The transitional care model (TCM): Hospital discharge screening criteria for high risk older adults. *Try This: Best Practices in Nursing Care of Older Adults, 26*. Retrieved from http://consultgerirn.org/uploads/File/trythis/try_this_26.pdf

Centers for Medicare and Medicaid Services. (2012). Readmission reduction program. Retrieved from http://cms.gov/Medicare/Medicare-Fee-for-Service-Payment/AcuteInpatientPPS/Readmissions-Reduction-Program.html/

Coleman, E. A., & Boult, C. E., on behalf of the American Geriatrics Society Health Care Systems Committee. (2003). Improving the quality of transitional care for persons with complex care needs. *Journal of the American Geriatrics Society, 51*(4), 556–557.

Coleman, E. A., Parry, C., Chalmers, S., & Min, S. J. (2006). The care transitions intervention: Results of a randomized controlled trial. *Archives of Internal Medicine, 166*, 1822–1828.

Forster, A. J., Murff, H. J., Peterson, J. F., Gandhi, T. K., & Bates, D. W. (2003). The incidence and severity of adverse events affecting patients after discharge from the hospital. *Annals of Internal Medicine, 138*, 161–167.

Foust, J. B., Naylor, M. D., Boling, P. A., & Capuzzo, K. A. (2005). Opportunities for improving post-hospital home medication management among older adults. *Home Health Care Services Quarterly, 24*(1), 101–122.

Foust, J. B., Vuckovic, N., & Henriquez, E. (2012). Hospital to home healthcare transition: Patient, caregiver and clinician perspectives. *Western Journal of Nursing Research, 34*(2), 194–212.

Graham, C. L., Ivey, S. L, & Neuhauser, L. (2009). From hospital to home: Assessing transitional care needs of vulnerable seniors. *Gerontologist, 49*(1), 23–33.

Holland, D. E., Harris, M. R., Leibson, C. L., Pankratz, V. S., & Kirchbaum, K. (2006). Development and validation of a screen for specialized discharge planning services. *Nursing Research, 55*(1), 62–71.

Jack, B. W., Chetty, V. K., Anthony, D., Greenwald, J. L., Sanchez, G. M., Johnson, A. E., …, Culpepper, L. (2009). A reengineered hospital discharge program to decrease rehospitalization: A randomized trial. *Annals of Internal Medicine, 150*, 178–187.

Joint Commission. (2010). *Advancing effective communication, cultural competence, and patient- and family-centered care: A roadmap for hospitals.* Oakbrook Terrace, IL: Author.

National Patient Safety Foundation. (2013). Ask me 3™. Retrieved from http://www.npsf.org/for-healthcare-professionals/programs/ask-me-3/

Naylor, M. D., Brooten, D., Campbell, R., Jacobsen, B. S., Mezey, M. D., Pauly, M. D., & Schwartz, J. S. (1999). Comprehensive discharge planning and home follow-up of hospitalized elders: A randomized clinical trial. *Journal of the American Medical Association, 281*, 613–620.

Naylor, M. D., Brooten, D. A., Campbell, R. L., Maislin, G., McCauley, K. M., & Schwartz, J. S. (2004). Transitional care of older adults hospitalized with heart failure: A randomized controlled trial, *Journal of the American Geriatrics Society, 52*, 675–684.

Rudak, S., Sandbœk, A., Lauritzen, T., & Christensen, B. (2005). Motivational interviewing: A systematic review and meta-analysis. *British Journal of General Practice, 55*, 305–312.

Transitional Care Model. (2008–2009). Retrieved from http://www.transitionalcare.info/

CHAPTER TEN

Physical Impairments to Communication

Janice B. Foust

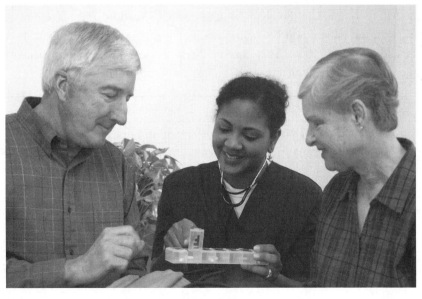

© Rob Marmion/ShutterStock, Inc.

■ CASE STUDY

A student nurse comes to the nurses' station on the rehabilitation floor of a skilled nursing facility looking for the clinical instructor. She is caring for Mr. G., a 74-year-old man, who has experienced a stroke and now has difficulty communicating verbally. Since his stroke, Mr. G. also has demonstrated difficulty controlling his emotions, and he is frequently angry with the nursing staff. Mr. G. is yelling so loudly at the student that he can be heard at the nurses' station down the hall. The student does not know what to do to help Mr. G. The student nurse acknowledges he knows Mr. G. is upset and leaves the room saying he is going to get some Mr. G. some help.

Introduction

How difficult it must be for anyone when he or she cannot communicate in the usual and familiar ways. Relaying messages through words and gestures is a complex process that becomes even more complicated when patients' usual abilities to communicate are compromised. Communication deficits might last for brief periods of time, such as during postoperative intubation, or they may result in permanent changes, such as when patients experience aphasia, hearing loss, or blindness. It is important to remember that each patient will try to adapt to the deficit to accommodate the changes in his or her situation. The nurse's role is to work with the patient and his or her abilities and maximize communication and independence (Box 10-1). This chapter discusses how physical impairments can hinder patients' communication and nursing implications.

Box 10-1	General Ways to Maximize Communication

- Learn the patient's preferred communication techniques—for example, sign language, hearing aid, or family member who interprets the meanings of words and gestures.
- Allow ample time and arrange for interpreters, if necessary.
- Place yourself at face level with the patient so that he or she can see your mouth and facial expressions.
- Speak distinctly and slowly, using a moderate tone.
- Provide paper and pencil or word boards to help the patient communicate, and provide written material to the patient as appropriate.

Speech and Language Deficits

Language is our basic way of communicating with the world—both receiving information and conveying our needs and feelings to others. Speech and language deficits may develop as part of the developmental process or as a result of illness. Such deficits may exist in receiving and/or expressing information and concerns. This section reviews three types of deficits: aphasia, hearing loss, and vision loss.

Aphasia

Nurses care for patients who experience aphasia, which is defined as "an absence or impairment of the ability to communicate by speech, writing or signs because of brain dysfunction" (Venes, 2013, p. 168), which includes several types of aphasia such as:

1. Expressive or motor aphasia: Words cannot be expressed or formed.
2. Receptive or sensory aphasia: Language is not understood.
3. Global aphasia: Includes both expressive and receptive deficits.

To develop the best communication strategies for patients with aphasia, the nurse needs to understand the individual patient, his or her specific abilities, and the medical condition contributing to aphasia. Accurate assessment of the type of aphasia and the methods used by the individual patient for communicating will help in planning the most appropriate nursing interventions (Box 10-2). Nurses work in collaboration with the healthcare team to develop an individualized plan. Team members may include primary and specialist physicians (e.g., neurologists),

---

Box 10-2 | Interventions for Communicating with Aphasic Patients

---

- Allow ample time for patients to formulate thoughts and receive information.
- Focus on the patient's abilities to communicate.
- Use touch, facial expressions, and sounds, as appropriate, and patient preferences.
- Supply alternative communication methods, such as word or picture boards, if current methods fail.
- Avoid prolonged conversations. Keep it short and to the point.
- Acknowledge the patient's efforts and use humor (as appropriate) to provide relaxation when communication becomes difficult.

---

occupational therapists, and speech therapists. Creating an individualized plan requires developing appropriate strategies to communicate that match the patient's strengths and abilities. For patients who have expressive aphasia, the team will need to identify efficient and effective ways for patients to express themselves.

Communicating with patients who have any type of aphasia requires nurses to be sensitive and convey respect for patients in ways that can be understood and appreciated by them. Patients who have experienced a stroke will likely benefit from multifaceted interventions to promote communication to meet their specific needs. For example, researchers have identified effective interventions with patients recovering from strokes (Poslawsky, Schuurmans, Lindeman, & Hadsteinsdóttir, 2010), including appropriate early screening for aphasia, speech-language therapy, task-specific interventions, use of augmented alternative means of communication such as alphabet boards, and use of computers. The authors emphasize the importance of close nurse–speech language therapist collaboration.

Another study described interactions between patients who had a stroke and nurses as they provided personal care (Sundin & Jansson, 2003). The authors described *co-creating* as a theme that represented the development of a nurse–patient relationship that emerged as care was provided. Conveying respect and use of nonverbal communication were evident in their descriptions. The nurses discussed the use of touch as a form of *silent dialogue*, which attended to the patient's needs and wishes. Similarly, they described situations when they used eye contact to assess the patient's response and readiness to do a task. One of the strategies they used to create a supportive atmosphere was the use of small talk that did not require patients to respond but allowed them to do so as they wished.

Hearing Loss

Hearing allows the listener not only to receive verbal messages, but also to interpret sounds in the environment. Hearing loss can be a result of the aging process or the result of trauma or illness or present at birth. Cues in the environment, such as a ringing phone or a honking car, might not be heard by a person with a hearing impairment, perhaps posing safety concerns. Relationships with others are affected by hearing loss as well, because the person with the hearing deficit might not only miss the words but also be unable to detect subtle changes in voice, such as pitch, tone, or volume.

Noise levels in the environment also affect the person's ability to hear and understand conversations. For example, it can be difficult for patients to hear the nurse when a roommate's television is on or nearby conversations are occurring in the hallway. In one study, older adults living in residential facilities experienced varying levels of concerns with their own hearing loss or hearing loss in others living in the facility (Pryce & Gooberman-Hill, 2012). The researchers found that background noise negatively affected older adults' participation in social activities. Music and televisions were commonly playing and some residents preferred it sometimes be turned off. They also described problems as including using the telephone or televisions, as well as expressed concern for other residents who did not hear well, and feelings of depression or helplessness among hearing-impaired individuals.

Assessment of hearing loss is important when planning nursing care. Knowing the age of onset, type of loss, use of aids, and medical conditions or circumstances is essential to planning appropriate interventions. For example, older adults may have cerumen (earwax) buildup that, if removed, would improve their hearing. Hearing loss in childhood may contribute to problems with learning to speak, learning in general, participating in social activities, and communicating with others. People with hearing and speech deficits may use sign language or use hearing aids as assistive devices to facilitate communication. Older people may have difficulty manipulating hearing aids or tiny batteries, and, as a result, may not wear them. At other times, older people with hearing loss may choose not to use their hearing aids because the aids amplify too many sounds, which makes it difficult to hear or discern conversations.

Nurses must be mindful of the patient's environment, pace of conversation, and tone of voice, and use face-face to communication whenever possible (Box 10-3). In the context of busy work environments, nurses should be sure to face patients so they may read the nurse's lips (if patients use this strategy) and more easily follow what is being said. Nurses working in outpatient settings may call patients with information or to remind them of office visits. In these situations, it would be helpful to have the patient repeat back the information and allow time for questions or clarifying the information. In some instances, it would be wise or necessary to follow up with written correspondence.

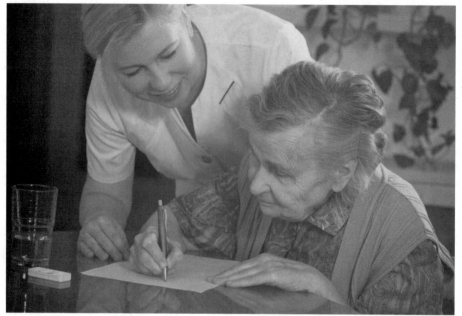

Nurses adapt their interactions to use the patient's preferred modes of communication.

Box 10-3	Interventions for Communicating with Patients with Hearing Loss

- Use the method that works best for your patient—hearing aid, sign language, written words, or adjusting the volume of your voice.
- Arrange for interpreters to explain the patient's methods of communicating, and refer the patient to an audiologist, if necessary.
- Help patients use hearing aids and assess whether the hearing aid is working properly.
- Speak in a moderate, even tone; do not yell.
- Face the patient when talking so that he or she can see movements of the mouth and facial expressions.
- Consult with a speech therapist and/or an audiologist to learn the best communication strategies for the individual patient.

Vision Loss

Vision loss or blindness cause communication deficits because patients may not be able to read written information or see nonverbal gestures, postures, and body language. Similar to patients with hearing loss, people with vision loss may feel isolated and vulnerable, especially when they are in an unfamiliar environment, such as a hospital setting. Older adults may experience age-related changes that contribute to vision loss and nursing implications (Whiteside, Wallhagen, & Pettengill, 2006). Normal vision changes often reduce older adults' vision, creating difficulty in accommodating changes in brightness and increasing sensitivity to glare. Strategies to help older adults with vision loss include increasing the contrast of written materials, using proper lighting and sunglasses, modifying the environment, and using assistive devices (e.g., magnifying glass) (Whiteside et al., 2006). It is very important that nurses work with the healthcare team to identify community resources that may provide information and assistance as people adjust to their vision loss.

Nurses need to assess the individual patient's vision loss, including the type of loss (light, shadows, complete), any types of aids used (e.g., Braille, cane, glasses), medical condition (e.g., cataracts, glaucoma), and circumstances leading to the vision loss and when the vision loss occurred (e.g., new diagnosis or chronic condition) (Box 10-4). The use of aids should be incorporated into the care plan

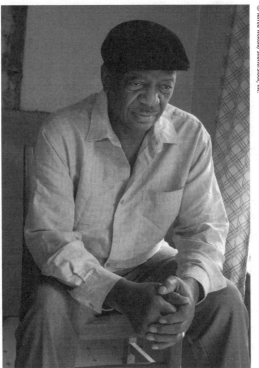

© Alfred Wekelo/ShutterStock, Inc.

Vision loss may impair communication and make patients feel isolated and vulnerable.

Box 10-4 Interventions for Communicating with Patients with Vision Loss

- Alert the patient when you approach and state your name.
- Do not speak loudly or overly enunciate.
- Orient the patient to the surroundings (e.g. call bell), mentioning furniture (or other barriers), steps, or changes in terrain in advance.
- Offer assistance to the patient who is navigating new surroundings.
- Ask other personnel to introduce themselves to the patient when they enter and leave the room.
- Explain procedures in advance so that the patient knows what to expect.
- Describe activities going on around the patient as well as direct nursing interventions.
- Tell the patient when you are leaving the room.
    - Consult colleagues (e.g. social worker, case manager) for information about community resources

---

so that patients can maintain their usual functioning and adapted abilities while receiving health care. Further referral to an ophthalmologist/optometrist may be necessary to optimize visual acuity. In addition, the nurse may work with the healthcare team to identify available community resources.

Sensory Deprivation in Intensive Care Settings

Intensive care units, emergency rooms, and recovery rooms can be strange and frightening environments for patients. Unfamiliar surroundings, noises, and equipment can be disorienting, and patients may also be in pain, intubated, or medicated—all of which may impair communication. It is important for nurses to provide explanations and reassurance in such bewildering settings to patients (Box 10-5). Nurses often orient the patients and their families to the environment, equipment, and what they may expect (e.g., routines) while patients are there. These conversations are repeated as needed as a strategy to reduce anxiety.

As described earlier, patients in high-acuity settings may experience multiple and sudden changes in their abilities to communicate. For example, an older adult may be intubated after cardiac surgery in an intensive care

---

Box 10-5 Interventions for Communicating with Patients in Intensive Care Settings

- Tell the patient your name and role before implementing any intervention.
- Speak as though the patient hears everything.
- Orient the patient frequently to the surroundings, explaining sights and sounds, date and time, and healthcare staff.
- Give explanations about procedures before they occur and explain different sights and sounds that the patient might experience.
- Provide information to the patient about his or her progress.
- Even if the patient cannot speak, carry on a one-way conversation.
    - Use eye contact and touch, as appropriate.
- Encourage the patient and/or family to display items that are meaningful to the patient, such as photographs or simple objects from home, as appropriate.
- Consult with speech therapists and others about strategies and potential use of augmented communication devices.

---

unit. Factors that may impair communication include age-related changes with hearing and vision, an inability to speak while intubated, and significant and unfamiliar background noises (e.g., numerous alarms and conversations). Nurses need to develop an individualized communication plan with the patient (see the evidence-based article identified at the end of this chapter) and family.

Another example of a setting that may create problems for patients with sensory deficits is the perioperative environment. In this situation, nurses can provide glasses, hearing aids, and other devices until the patient receives anesthesia for surgery, and then return these items as soon as the patient is sufficiently alert. Frequent assessments of the patient's mental status are essential to determine the patient's needs and direct adjustments to nursing interventions. These assessments will be more accurate when patients are using any of their assistive devices (e.g., hearing aids) when possible. Postanesthesia care units may be windowless and full of strange sounds and constant light. Nurses need to introduce themselves; remind patients of the date, time, and reason why they are in the postanesthesia care unit; and explain the environment sounds and procedures.

Summary

Physical impairments affect patients' ability to communicate with nurses by altering their abilities to receive and/or express information. Patients often adapt and convey their messages regardless of the type, reason, or duration of the physical impairment. Nurses are in a unique position to identify and implement or support patients' preferred methods of communicating with others. Nurses work with the healthcare team to facilitate services and make referrals to help patients with deficits communicate with healthcare providers.

Case Study Resolution

Student: "I don't know what to do. I have tried to find out what he wants but he just keeps yelling at me. What am I doing wrong?"

Instructor: "Let's go see Mr. G., and maybe we can figure it out."

Student: (In Mr. G.'s room) Introduces his instructor and says, "Mr. G., we want to make you more comfortable. How can we help you?" Mr. G. shakes his head, yells again, and points at the bed.

Student: "It seems that something is wrong with the bed or bedding. Would you help me roll him over and I'll smooth out the sheets. Mr. G., we are going to fix the sheets."

As they roll Mr. G. on his side, the student finds the remote control to the television under his sacrum. The skin around the area is indented from the remote.

Mr. G. gives a relaxed sigh and reaches over and grasps and shakes the student's hand, indicating his gratitude.

Website

Lighthouse International

This organization provides useful and helpful information about low vision or blindness for people in the community and professionals.

http://www.lighthouse.org/

Evidence-Based Article

Happ, M. B., Garrett, K., Thomas, D. D., Tate, J., George, E., Houze, M., ..., & Sereika, S. (2011). Nurse–patient communication interactions in the intensive care unit. *American Journal of Critical Care, 20,* e28–e40.

This study observed nurse–patient interactions in an intensive care unit using video recordings. Nurses initiated most communication with patients. Eye contact was among the most common positive communication strategies along with use of gesturing and asking open-ended questions. However, a lack of eye contact was the most frequent negative communication behavior by nurses. In a majority of interactions, patients did not view the communication as difficult or saw it as entailing little difficulty. Nonverbal gestures were the most common strategy used by patients communicating with the nurses. Communication about pain was less successful than other areas, which the authors identified as important areas for more attention. In addition, increased use of assistive communication devices was one of the authors' recommendations.

References

Poslawsky, I. E., Schuurmans, M. J., Lindeman, E., & Hadsteinsdóttir, T. B., on behalf of the Rehabilitation Guide Stroke Working Group. (2010). A systematic review of nursing rehabilitation of stroke patients with aphasia. *Journal of Clinical Nursing, 19*, 17–32.

Pryce, H., & Gooberman-Hill, R. (2012). "There's a hell of a noise": Living with a hearing loss in residential care. *Age and Ageing, 41*, 40–46.

Sundin, K., & Jansson, L. (2003). 'Understanding and being understood' as a creative caring phenomenon – in care of patients with stroke and aphasia. *Journal of Clinical Nursing, 12*, 107–116.

Venes, D. (Ed.). (2013). *Taber's cyclopedic medical dictionary*. Philadelphia: F. A. Davis.

Whiteside, M. M., Wallhagen, M. I., & Pettengill, E. (2006). Sensory impairment in older adults: Part 2: Vision loss. *American Journal of Nursing, 106*(11), 52–61.

CHAPTER ELEVEN

Talking with Children: Working with Families

Esther Seibold, DNSc, RN

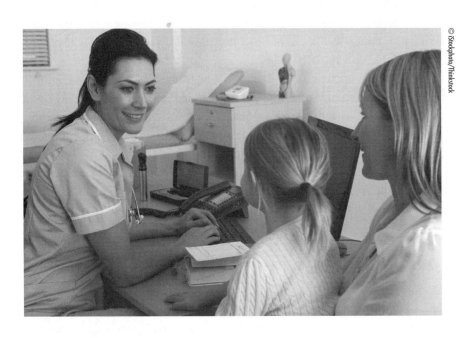

■ **CASE STUDY**

Maria is a 9-year-old female who is admitted to a pediatric teaching hospital for reconstructive surgery. She has a history of a complex medical syndrome and numerous previous admissions. She has traveled from another country to this medical center with her parents. The family has been in the hospital for approximately 1 month. Maria is very depressed and is refusing to cooperate with dressing changes and other procedures. She states that she just wants to go home. The parents, who speak only a little English, are frustrated because they have been away from their home, their family, and their other children for a long time. The nurse is trying to communicate with the family about discharge care for their daughter and transition to home but is having difficulty engaging the parents.

Background

Care of children in the healthcare setting, whether acute care or community based, is premised on the concept of family-centered care. Not only does the nurse care for the child, but he or she also cares for the family. In fact, when caring for a child with an illness, the family—rather than just the patient—is the unit of care. Family-centered care emphasizes family–professional collaboration and communication, as well as respecting the cultural diversity of individual families (Bowden & Greenberg, 2010).

This framework has several implications that affect communication with children and their families. First, parents are included in a wide range of conversations with the entire team of healthcare professionals who are caring for their child. Second, specific communication skills will require appropriate interactions and exchanges with both the child in question and his or her family members. The nurse will need to utilize different communication patterns when speaking with the child, as opposed to speaking with his or her parents. Therefore, communication with children and with parents will be addressed separately.

Communicating with Children

Communication with children should always take place at a developmentally appropriate level (Table 11-1). It is important to remember that developmental age is not always the same as chronological age. Thus, when assessing how to

Table 11-1 Communicating with Children

Age	Developmental Considerations	Useful Techniques
Infant (0–12 months)	Trust versus mistrust Stranger anxiety Nonverbal communication Beginning verbalization	Establish rapport through touch, feeding, simple communication. Primary information exchange is with parents.
Toddler (12–36 months)	Vocabulary increases from 10 to several hundred words Increasing sentence complexity Increasing ability to comprehend and follow commands Separation anxiety	Use simple commands; use familiar terms. Encourage family presence to minimize stress. Establish rapport through play, both physical and imaginary.
Preschooler (3–6 years)	Can articulate experiences such as pain, as well as emotions Awareness of body and body parts, as well as sense of self	Use play, stories, and books. Be honest. Use family terms for concepts such as pain and body parts.
School age (6–12 years)	Increasing language and conceptual comprehension Knowledge of body parts and functions	Use writing, drawing, storytelling, and multimedia resources to convey relevant information.
Adolescence (12–18 years)	Increasing independence Privacy Confidentiality Broad range of emotional maturity to make decisions Consent versus assent	Include adolescents in planning and decision making.

talk with a child, and especially one with special needs, the nurse must determine what the child is able to understand and at what level the child can communicate his or her needs and condition. Remember that as the child's language skills are developing, receptive skills typically precede expressive skills, so children may understand words about pain and emotions but may not be able to articulate their own experiences.

Developmentally Appropriate Communication

Infants (0–12 months): Respond to tone of voice, familiar voices and sounds, touch; communicate by crying. From 1 month to approximately 6 months, infants will allow strangers to touch and hold them. From 6 to 12 months, infants will not go to unfamiliar individuals, due to stranger anxiety. The nurse should engage with the infant to establish a sense of trust. Interactions such as appropriate comforting, feeding, and other caregiving activities will facilitate developing a relationship with the infant.

Toddlers (12–36 months): Progress from understanding words and simple commands to following more complex thoughts and commands. Toddlers are progressively able to articulate words, then phrases, and finally simple sentences. They retain information for only short periods of time, so teaching should be in simple language and close to the time of intervention or procedure. Nurses should use family-preferred words to describe pain, body parts, or other actions or objects. Use dolls and picture books to help convey concepts.

Preschoolers (3–5 years): Children from ages 3 to 5 years have a greater mastery of vocabulary and can articulate both their experiences and their feelings. They can follow instructions that are presented in simple, straightforward language. Use of play, stories, and books will help to convey or elicit relevant information. Nurses should be honest and use simple and family-preferred terms. Preschoolers may be given choices when appropriate.

School age (6–12 years): Children from 6 to 12 years develop not only extensive expressive language skills but also greater comprehension skills. In addition, this is the age of logic and reason. Children in this age group can understand more about their bodies, as well as the physical and psychological impact of various procedures. Children can be helped to express their feelings with techniques such as third-party storytelling, writing, or drawing. Nurses should answer all questions directly, using diagrams, illustrations, books, and video materials.

Adolescents (12–18 years): Teens may be able to understand the terminology of a disease or procedure but may not have the emotional maturity to comprehend the consequences of these processes. Nurses should respect their need for privacy and confidentiality as appropriate. The adolescent should be included in decision making and planning as much as possible, always making sure to include the family in the process as necessary.

Nonverbal Communication

In addition to words, many types of nonverbal communication are used to communicate. In some cases, lack of recognition of these behaviors may lead to miscommunication that interferes with nurse–patient interactions. When working with children, the nurse should be aware of the following nonverbal patterns that he or she might inadvertently employ:

- Facial expressions: may imply interest, neutrality, or anxiety.
- Body posture: sitting face to face will indicate friendliness, while body tension may indicate anger.
- Gestures such as leg shaking or finger tapping: may indicate anxiety or frustration. The nurse's use of the "hands on hips" gesture may indicate authority and can intimidate both a child and the parent.
- Eye contact: indicates interest and honesty and is useful in engaging both children and parents.

The nurse should also attempt to interpret the body language of the child and/or parents, thereby adding to his or her understanding of the family members' state of coping. Some aspects of nonverbal communication are culturally based and will influence how a family member interacts with the nurse and other staff, including personal space and distance, touching, and handshaking.

Finally, the nurse should be familiar with how to establish trust and rapport with a child. Children, especially when they are experiencing stress or not feeling well, may not want to interact with strangers, particularly when there are many new people who want to talk with or examine them. Therefore the nurse has to establish a therapeutic relationship as part of the child's care, often by first communicating with the parents. This lets the child see that the nurse is not threatening. Play is also another method of engaging with the child and establishing rapport.

Communicating with Family Members

In addition to talking with children, the nurse will communicate directly with family members. The nurse will need to perform an assessment of family structure to identify the various roles and relationships of the family members and determine who will be staying with the child and making decisions during hospitalization. Family assessment should also include evaluation of the level of stress and coping mechanisms of the family. These factors can influence how well the family manages the hospitalization experience, and this information will provide the nurse with clues about effective communication strategies.

As a patient advocate, it will often be the nurse's responsibility to help the family understand all the medical information that is being given to them. In general, nurses should minimize the use of technical language and jargon and try to respect linguistic and cultural factors. The nurse should elicit from the parents specific terminology used in the family to talk about such concepts as pain (e.g., "owie," "boo-boo," "hurt") and body parts (family terms for genitals, bowel and bladder elimination, and so on).

Families can be resources regarding many kinds of useful information about their children, including their daily routines, preferences, sleep patterns, and more. Interviewing parents about these details enables the nurse to plan the child's care and daily routine more effectively and minimize disruptions.

Some general considerations for talking with parents include the following:

1. Listen genuinely to the parents' concerns about their child's care.
2. Show respect for the parents.
3. Maintain a nonjudgmental approach.
4. Assist the parents in identifying their own and their child's needs and priorities.
5. Engage the parents in caring for their child in whatever aspects they feel comfortable.
6. Be available to answer questions as they arise.

Summary

The key components of communication with children and their families include consideration of family-centered care, developmentally appropriate communication, and cultural diversity and language awareness. By following the guidelines described in this chapter, the nurse should be able to successfully establish good communication with pediatric patients and their families.

Case Study Resolution

There are several key factors to consider regarding Maria and her family. These include language and cultural issues, being far away from family and usual support systems, and the needs of a 9-year-old child. The fact that Maria and her family have come from another country for treatment has numerous implications. First, we know that the parents speak only a little English, and we have no information regarding Maria's fluency in this language. Even if we assume that Maria can communicate her needs adequately in English, it requires significant effort for a non-native speaker to communicate effectively, especially in a stressful situation such as hospitalization.

Second, both Maria and her parents are far away from their usual family, friends, and support systems. At 9 years of age, Maria likely misses her friends and usual activities. Issues such as returning to school and special accommodations will have to be addressed. The parents do not have regular access to their community of friends, family, and perhaps spiritual resources, and they must cope with language as well as other barriers on their own. In addition, discharge instructions will have to be shared with their local community upon their return, and local customs and resources may differ from those available in the United States.

The family should receive both verbal and written instructions, and this information should be clear enough to be translated into comparable activities, treatments, and medications that are available in their home country. A translator will likely be required to assist with this process. Aspects of culturally competent care should be part of the nursing staff's preparation to work with patients and families from diverse backgrounds.

Websites

The Challenge of Communicating with Pediatric Patients, American Academy of Orthopedic Surgeons.
http://www.aaos.org/news/aaosnow/feb09/clinical5.asp

American Academy of Pediatrics, www.aap.org, offers articles on pediatrician and resident communication with children.

HealthyChildren.org, a website associated with the American Academy of Pediatrics, offers many articles on parent–children communication.

Evidence-Based Article

Greydanus, D. E., & Kaplan, G. (2012). Strategies to improve medication adherence in youths. *Psychiatric Times, 29*(7), 14–16.

This article addresses the role of limited communication as a factor influencing nonadherence to medication regimens for adolescents with psychiatric disorders. Providers are encouraged to take the time to establish good rapport with the patient, engaging the patient at his or her cognitive level, providing a warm and accepting environment, establishing trust between the clinician and patient, engaging in shared decision making, having the patient consent to treatment, maintaining confidentiality, and utilizing newer technologies such as email and texting to improve medication adherence in adolescents.

References

Bowden, V., & Greenberg, C. (2010). *Children and their families: The continuum of care* (2nd ed.). Philadelphia, PA: Wolters Kluwer Health/Lippincott Williams & Wilkins.

Additional References

Ball, J. W., Bindler, R. C., & Cowan, K. J. (2010). *Child health nursing* (2nd ed.). Hoboken, NJ: Pearson Education.

El-Amouri, S., & O'Neill, S. (2011). Supporting cross-cultural communication and culturally competent care in the linguistically and culturally diverse hospital settings of UAE. *Contemporary Nurse, 19*(2), 240–255.

Hockenberry, M., & Wilson, D. (2010). *Wong's nursing care of infants and children* (9th ed.). Cambridge, MA: Elsevier Health Sciences.

Kyle, T., & Carmen, S. (2012). *Essentials of pediatric nursing* (2nd ed.). Philadelphia, PA: Lippincott Williams & Wilkins.

Pilliteri, A. (2007). *Maternal and child health nursing: Care of the childbearing and childrearing family* (5th ed.). Philadelphia, PA: Lippincott Williams & Wilkins.

CHAPTER TWELVE

Nurses as Educators: Simulation, Communication, and Patient Care

Judith Healey Walsh, EdDc, MS, RN
Jennifer Mardin Small, MSN, RN

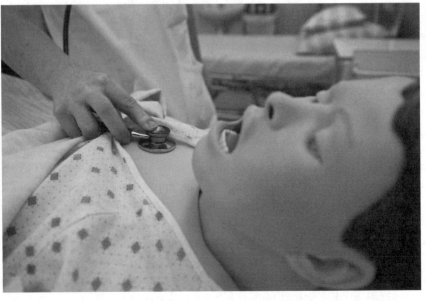

■ **CASE STUDY**

Maria Cavaro is a 24-year-old, English-speaking, Latina female on a postpartum unit who had a vaginal delivery of a baby girl 1 hour ago. Mrs. Cavaro had an uncomplicated but quick delivery and did not receive any pain medications or epidural during her delivery. The nurse is completing a postpartum physical assessment on Mrs. Cavaro. When she removes the blankets to examine her perineal area, the nurse finds a large pool of blood between the patient's legs. The nurse, upon seeing the large amount of blood, states, "Oh my God, that's a lot of blood." Mrs. Cavaro's husband leaps up from his chair and looks stunned. He says to the nurse, "Is she going to be alright?" The nurse reassures him by saying, "She is going to be fine." The nurse explains that she is going to call the physician to update her on his wife's bleeding. The nurse pages the physician; when she answers, the nurse states, "Mrs. Cavaro is bleeding excessively. Can you come right away?"

Introduction

As evidenced in other chapters, communication is a complex process, yet it is a core component of safe, patient-centered, high-quality nursing practice. Although communication can be read about and discussed in isolation, in reality during a clinical encounter communication occurs on many levels and within a specific context. In one clinical encounter, communication will occur between several dyads, including nurse–patient, nurse–family member, nurse–nurse, and nurse–physician. Each interaction requires a different style of communication, yet collectively such interactions can occur in a "rapid-fire" fashion, creating a challenging and stressful situation for both nursing students and nurses. In addition, the need to communicate occurs in a context where the nurse is always performing other cognitive and psychomotor activities. For example, while the nurse is inserting a catheter, the patient may be asking if it will be painful, while the family member is questioning why the patient needs it, while the nursing student is struggling to maintain sterile technique. Particularly for the student and novice nurse, it may be difficult to perform assessments, procedures, and clinical reasoning while also responding to questions and concerns from the patient and/or family member.

Communication failures are the leading cause of sentinel events and unintentional patient harm (Leonard, Graham, & Bonacum, 2004). Therefore, nursing students need practice in integrating effective communication strategies with patients, family members, and other health team members into the complexity of patient care situations. Simulation—an innovative teaching method—provides a learning environment that supports this practice. This chapter presents a brief overview of simulation and the lessons learned about nursing students' struggles with communication skills. The lessons and examples were culled from 5 years of experience facilitating hundreds of simulation sessions for students who were enrolled in medical–surgical, maternity, and pediatric clinical courses.

Simulation

Simulation provides a unique modality for experiential learning and has been found to integrate theory and practice while promoting acquisition of the technical, critical thinking, and communication skills needed to provide competent, safe patient care (Gaba, 2004; Seropian, 2003). The National Council of State Boards of Nursing (NCSBN, 2005) defines simulation as an educational process, which provides a learning experience that imitates the working environment and requires that the learner demonstrate procedural techniques, decision making, effective communication, and critical thinking. High-fidelity simulation uses human patient simulators (HPS), which are computerized manikins that mimic human physiology and allow the students to perform sophisticated assessments and interventions. The simulations occur in an environment that mirrors the realism of the clinical setting, including the use of authentic medical equipment and supplies. The simulation is interactive as students, usually working in groups of four, assume specific roles, and the faculty member in the control room becomes the voice of the patient and the physician (if called). Patient safety, communication, teamwork, clinical assessment and judgment, and psychomotor skills are threaded through every simulation.

High-fidelity simulation as an educational strategy has three distinct phases: presimulation (preparation phase), the actual simulation phase, and the postsimulation, debriefing phase. Each phase includes multiple steps and responsibilities (Rhodes & Curran, 2005). For the preparation phase, we give students a prep packet that provides an overview of the simulation; brief information about the patient, medications, procedures, and course content to review; and information on SBAR, a standardized communication tool used in many healthcare settings to improve intraprofessional and interprofessional communication (see Chapter 18 for more information on SBAR). SBAR stands for situation (S), background (B), assessment (A), and recommendation (R). This gives the nurse a structure and predictable format to use when communicating with a physician, during handoff to another nurse, or when transferring patients to other areas of care. This format prompts the nurse to be focused and concise in their communication and to use critical thinking to make recommendations about possible solutions or areas that need follow-up (Leonard et al., 2004). Just prior to the simulation, we review the process and what to expect, assign the roles, and orient the students to the patient room and equipment. We have found the preparation phase to be vitally important to both student performance and learning. Students who have reviewed all the prep material, know where supplies and equipment are located, and know how to use them are more confident and less anxious, are better able to perform procedures, and have the energy and ability to attend to clinical reasoning and communication issues.

The roles usually include a primary nurse and a secondary nurse. The primary nurse is the nurse assigned to the patient and is ultimately responsible for the care. The secondary nurse is a colleague who has stepped in to assist with the patient. Having these two roles allows the students to practice and assess their intraprofessional communication and teamwork. We always include a family member or significant other so that students can practice their interactions with family members, who may be highly emotional and expressing many questions and concerns. This helps students learn how to respond respectfully and effectively, and when and how to set gentle limits. The typical fourth role is the observer recorder, who remains quiet throughout the simulation but is document-ing all aspects of the care rendered, including communication and any elements missed by the nurses. As mentioned earlier, the faculty member assumes the role of the patient and physician. In this capacity we are able to formulate ques-tions and concerns, which we hope will elicit certain responses from the student. In addition, as the voice of the physician, we can vary our responses based on the student's ability to communicate the essential information in a clear and succinct manner.

The second phase involves the actual simulation case. Each simulation case has clear and specific learning objectives, and one always pertains to effective communication. During the simulation, the student must determine how to address multiple and competing demands. For example, after making introductions, the student usually begins his or her assessment, and the faculty member may have the patient ask a challenging question requiring the student to determine what to do. Additionally, the patient's status may begin to deteriorate so that the student is trying to either further assess to find the cause or intervene to alleviate the cause when the family member becomes extremely concerned, emotional, or inquisitive regarding the status of the patient. The student must determine how to prioritize the patient's needs and family members' concerns and communicate respectfully and effectively within this context.

Within a simulated scenario, the faculty member can observe and evaluate a student's verbal and nonverbal communication skills. Simulation scenarios are oftentimes recorded and reviewed during the debriefing, which allows the students to observe and evaluate their own verbal and nonverbal communication skills and identify areas that need to be improved.

The third and final phase of simulation involves the debriefing session, where much of the learning actually occurs. This session takes place immediately following the actual case and is facilitated by the faculty member, who guides students through reflection on and discussion of their individual and team performance, including communication. The faculty facilitator can often make suggestions or encourage the students to devise alternative ways in which they could have communicated or ways they could have phrased statements in a more effective manner. Watching the recording is "eye opening" for students, who at times are shocked at their verbal and nonverbal communication. The reflections provide powerful insights into the need for ongoing skill development in communication strategies and motivation to practice and refine these skills at clinical. Students are always very engaged in the discussion around communication and appreciate the opportunity that simulation offers for practicing and evaluating their communication skills. Most importantly, high-fidelity simulation as an innovative pedagogy has been found to provide a safe environment for educating nursing students without risk to human life and to assist learners in transferring knowledge and skills, including communication skills, to actual clinical practice (Jeffries & Rogers, 2007; Morgan, Cleave-Hogg, Desousa, & Lam-McCulloch, 2006).

Communication Lessons Learned

For ease of understanding, we have categorized our observations and lesson learned according to the communication dyad.

Nurse–Patient

VERBAL AND NONVERBAL OVER-REACTION

As can be seen in the case study cited at the beginning of this chapter, students struggle with how to respond when during their assessment they see something of major concern. They are unable to filter their immediate reaction both verbally and nonverbally. During debriefing, when students realize how they responded, they are shocked and dismayed. They can see how their communication caused an increase in stress and anxiety in both the patient and the family member. Students and faculty discuss how to avoid this by developing a "poker face," taking a deep breath, and thinking about a better way to verbally respond, such as "I see that you have some bleeding. This can happen after a delivery, and there are some things that I can to do stop it. I am also going to call your doctor to update her." Students have found this discussion to be extremely helpful, and they begin anticipating possible reactions and practice developing communication skills that convey the most appropriate and effective response.

RELAYING TOO MUCH INFORMATION

Frequently, when faced with a patient's questions about his or her condition, students' inexperience, anxiety, and uncertainty about how to respond lead them to relay too much information. Subsequently, the patient's reaction and further probing becomes problematic, increasing the student's anxiety.

For example, during a maternity simulation case, a pregnant woman who has preeclampsia asks the nursing students why they are administering magnesium sulfate. Many students respond by saying, "Your blood pressure is very high and we want to prevent a seizure, which could harm you and the baby." In response, the faculty member, as the voice of the patient, will express anxiety about the word "seizure" and ask if the baby is going to die; the students hesitate because they are unsure how best to respond. Students struggle with, on the one hand, how to provide information that they think a patient has a right to know and, on the other hand, how to protect the patient from unnecessary anxiety and upset that could negatively impact the patient's condition. This is a challenging skill that only improves with experience and practice. During the debriefing, students and the facilitator discuss this type of challenge and practice different ways that the student could respond, still being honest with the patient but also avoiding increasing the patient's stress level.

PROVIDING FALSE REASSURANCE

Students also typically respond to patients' questions and concerns about their health status with false reassurance. In a case where the patient was admitted with chest pain and is told that she has had a myocardial infarction (MI), she becomes very upset and asks the nursing student if she is going to die. Students' initial reaction is to allay the patient's fear and anxiety by responding, "No, you are not going to die; you'll be fine." But the patient's condition deteriorates in the scenario, and she goes into cardiac arrest. In the debriefing, students will discuss how it seemed natural to reassure the patient, but they realize that it is not helpful or ethical to provide this reassurance when it is uncertain how the patient's condition will progress. It is more honest and appropriate to respond by simply stating, "We are going to provide the best care possible."

IGNORING QUESTIONS OR CONCERNS

In high-stress situations when the patient's condition is deteriorating and the patient expresses concern or asks a question, the nursing student frequently ignores the question. Typically, students do this because they are distracted with their own thinking as they try to process the situation and intervene effectively. At other times students ignore the question because they are uncertain about how they should respond. We have also seen that the students ignore questions or concerns on the part of the patient when the two nurses are trying to solve a medication calculation together. Often their back is turned and they are completely disengaged from the patient. When students observe this behavior, they realize how uncaring it appears to the patient, although that was not their intention. Students then discuss that more effective communication would involve acknowledging that the patient has a question or concern and that they will address it once they have completed their assessment or intervention.

Nurse–Family

CONFIDENTIALITY ISSUES

Students frequently share too much personal information in front of a family member without first asking the patient if it is okay to discuss the patient's health status. They make the assumption that, because they are related, any information can be provided in front of the family member. In debriefing, the discussion includes how important it is to get patients' verbal consent to discuss their health state in front of any visitors.

IGNORING QUESTIONS OR CONCERNS

During simulations, nursing students were observed ignoring family members' questions and concerns. This was specifically noted in a pediatric simulation that involved a child with a tracheostomy that needed to be suctioned. Many students had difficulty interacting with the patient's mother as she expressed concerns and asked questions about her son's condition because they were distracted or focused on the psychomotor task of suctioning. The students either did not feel comfortable or were unsure how to explain to the mother that they needed to concentrate on the procedure and then would respond to their questions. Students struggle with how and when it is appropriate to delay answering questions.

IMPATIENT RESPONSE

Students have also demonstrated that they can become irritated with the questioning from a family member. We have seen students raise their voice, respond rudely, demonstrate their frustration nonverbally (facial expression, posture, eye-rolling), or ask a family member to leave when the family member is simply showing concern and looking for explanation about their loved one's condition. In debriefing, the student can reflect on their behavior and determine why they communicated in this manner and how it would impact both the patient and family member. They usually are insightful and realize that the source of this behavior was their anxiety or inability to address the patient's needs and respond to the family member's question at the same time.

Nurse–Nurse

NO COMMUNICATION

During some simulated scenarios, the two nurses would not communicate at all. In some instances, the two would work alongside each other but neglect to share the information that each had gathered with the other, making for fragmented care of the patient. For example, one nurse might assess the lung sounds of the patient who is short of breath but not share with the other nurse that she auscultated crackles bilaterally. If the two nurses did not share information and work as a team, it was impossible for them work together to discover what was wrong with the patient and how best to intervene.

In other cases, the primary nurse would assume total responsibility for the care of the patient while the secondary nurse stood idle in the room. During this scenario, it was evident that there was a lack of a team effort to provide care to the patient and the primary nurse did not receive the benefit of idea sharing and group critical thinking to determine the next course of action.

In these cases, the communication with the patient, family member, and physician were all negatively impacted by a lack of teamwork. In debriefing, students are often able to see how the lack of teamwork affected their communication ability and style, and ultimately the quality of care provided to the patient.

INAPPROPRIATE COMMUNICATION

Some simulated scenarios are higher in stress level than others because of the learning level of the student or the objectives of the scenario. For example, a scenario used for final-semester senior nursing students results in a patient nearly going into respiratory arrest from the administration of intravenous morphine for pain. Due to the high stress and critical nature of the patient, the nurses in the scenario often demonstrate inappropriate communication with one another. We have witnessed students yelling or getting frustrated with each other or even bullying each other when they feel the scenario is not going well. Rather than working as a team, their stress and anxiety are taken out on each other. In debriefing, students are often surprised at their behavior or voice tone in the scenario and realize that in stressful environments they need to learn how to decrease and not misdirect their anxiety.

Nurse–Physician
PREMATURE COMMUNICATION

Frequently students panic when they believe that a patient's condition has changed or is deteriorating and call a physician too soon. They call for help or to report a finding without first completing the necessary assessment or information gathering, which actually results in delayed treatment of the patient. As the information is incomplete, the physician or care provider will end the phone call by instructing the nurse to call back when she or he has completed the patient assessment and organized all the pertinent information. When this is discussed or viewed in debriefing, the students can see how this behavior affects getting the necessary help for their patient. It is often evident that several additional minutes, which might be crucial in a fast-deteriorating patient, are wasted when the phone call is made too early. In addition, students are reminded of the importance and given the opportunity to practice their communication organization skills using the standardized SBAR format.

DISORGANIZED COMMUNICATION

When dealing with a stressful situation (as in the case study), nurses are often so anxious and overly focused on wanting the physician to come and assist that they are disorganized and leave out major identifying information about themselves and their patient. That is, key components of the SBAR communication are omitted. This leads to frustration for the physician or care provider, who then has to ask multiple questions or probe to get needed information about what is happening with the patient to determine the most immediate course of action.

TOO MUCH INFORMATION

In contrast, students can not be sufficiently concise and targetted in their interactions and communication with a physician. Doctors and nurses have very different communication styles: Physicians are concise and "to the point," whereas nurses are more narrative and want to "paint the big picture." In simulation, we have observed students giving excessive amounts of information as opposed to focusing on what is actually relevant to the current situation about which they are calling. The students struggle to determine what is most important; moreover, due to inexperience in communicating with physicians, they provide everything they know about a patient. For example, the students relay to the physician a history of glaucoma for a patient who is in pulmonary edema from a blood transfusion. Not being able to understand the value of brevity in an interaction with a physician can lead to mistreatment or delayed treatment of the patient.

TIMID COMMUNICATION

Because of a perceived power difference or difference in hierarchy between themselves and a physician, students can be too timid in their interactions with physicians. We have seen nurses delay calling a physician out of fear or because they do not feel empowered enough to insist that a physician come immediately to evaluate a patient when the physician expresses any resistance. Through reflection in debriefing, students are encouraged again to use the SBAR format, which will empower them to feel capable of providing clear and compelling evidence that will convince the physician to come and evaluate the patient without further coaxing by the nurse.

Case Study Resolution

The case study illuminates some typical communication errors made by nursing students, as observed during simulation. First, the student does not filter her reaction to seeing the postpartum hemorrhage. Her emotive response creates stress and anxiety in the patient and her husband. When the husband expresses his fear and asks if his wife will be alright, the student then communicates a false reassurance, as she cannot guarantee that the patient will be fine. The student then quickly calls the physician but does not use SBAR to provide all the pertinent information in an orderly manner and also reports that the patient is bleeding excessively, which would probably scare the patient and her husband.

The benefit of simulation is that the student could observe and reflect on the effects of her verbal and nonverbal communication. In addition, she would receive feedback from her peers and the facilitator, and be able to discuss more effective methods of communicating with the patient, family member, and the physician. These newly learned methods could then be used in the future in clinical settings.

Summary

Effective communication is essential to the provision of safe, high-quality, patient-centered care. Within a clinical encounter communication can occur at several different levels including nurse–patient, nurse–family member, nurse–nurse, and nurse–physician, with each interaction requiring different approaches to communication. In addition, nurses must communicate while they are also performing assessment, technical, and procedural functions. As communication failures are a root cause of many adverse clinical events, nursing students need opportunities to practice and gain competence in communication skills within the complex context of clinical care. Simulation provides a learning environment whereby nursing students can perform and evaluate their communication skills within a safe setting that mimics the challenges found in a clinical encounter. During the postsimulation debriefing students can reflect on the appropriateness of their communication with the patient, the family member, another nurse, and the physician, and as indicated, identify and discuss more effective communication techniques.

Evidence-Based Article

O'Shea, E. R., Pagano, M., Campbell, S. H., & Caso, G. (2013). A descriptive analysis of nursing student communication behaviors. *Clinical Simulation in Nursing, 9*(1), e5–e12.

This article describes a pilot study examining student nurses' communication behaviors during a maternal–child health simulation. The sample consisted of 55 senior nursing students from a baccalaureate program who were enrolled in an obstetrics or pediatrics clinical course. These students had engaged in approximately 15 or more simulations in prior courses. The simulations were audio and video recorded and independently reviewed by two maternal–child health nursing faculty, one physician assistant, and one graduate student from the Department of Communication. The goal of the video review was to determine whether researchers working independently could identify health communication behaviors that could affect patient care. The findings suggested that all of the researchers were able to identify a wide variety of health communication behaviors, but the communication authors were able to provide some specific insights into the students' verbal and nonverbal cues that the other researchers could not. The results suggested that using a multidisciplinary approach, including communication researchers, in simulation studies aimed at assessing communication skills is ideal.

References

Gaba, D. M. (2004). The future vision of simulation in health care. *Quality and Safety in Healthcare, 13*(Suppl. 1), i2–i10.

Jeffries, P. R., & Rogers, K. J. (2007). Theoretical framework for simulation design. In P. R. Jeffries (Ed.), *Simulation in nursing education*, (pp. 21–33). New York: National League for Nursing.

Leonard, M., Graham, S., & Bonacum, D. (2004). The human factor: The critical importance of effective teamwork and communication in providing safe care. *Quality and Safety in Healthcare, 13*(Suppl. 1), i85–i90.

Morgan, P. J., Cleave-Hogg, D., Desousa, S., & Lam-McCulloch, J. (2006). Applying theory to practice in undergraduate education using high fidelity simulation. *Medical Teacher, 28*(1), 10–14.

National Council of State Boards of Nursing. (2005). Clinical instruction in prelicensure nursing programs. Retrieved from http://www.ncsbn.org/Final_Clinical_Instr_Pre_Nsg_programs.pdf

Rhodes, M. L., & Curran, C. (2005). Use of the human patient simulator to teach clinical judgment skills in a baccalaureate nursing program. *CIN: Computers, Informatics, Nursing. 23*(5), 256–262.

Seropian, M. A. (2003). General concepts in full-scale simulation: Getting started. *Anesthesia and Analgesia, 97*(6), 1695–1705.

Difficult Communication

CHAPTER THIRTEEN

Communicating About Sexual Health Needs

Teri Aronowitz, PhD, FNP-BC

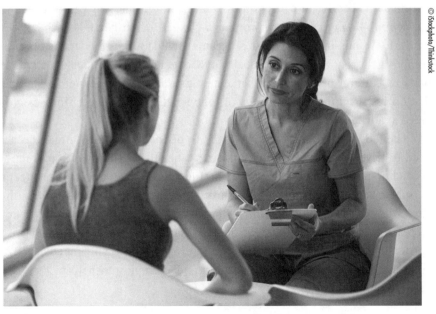

© iStockphoto/Thinkstock

■ CASE STUDY

L.S. and W.N. were high school sweethearts but went separate ways after graduation. Each found a new partner and had a family. After many years, L.S. lost her husband to heart disease and W.N. lost his wife to cancer. They reunited after moving to the same independent living center. After a lifetime apart, they easily rekindled their romance and after a 6-month courtship, they married. Both L.S. and W.N. have significant health problems. L.S., now 64, has had rheumatoid arthritis since her early 40s; her disease progressed rapidly, and she now uses a scooter to get around. She is independent in activities of daily living (ADLs) but does not drive. W.N., who is 65, smoked until 5 years ago, when he quit after experiencing a myocardial infarction (MI). He has significant chronic obstruction pulmonary disease (COPD) and uses continuous O_2. After losing 100 pounds, he has now begun having spontaneous erections.

Introduction

Generally speaking, healthcare professionals are not prepared to address the sexual health needs of their clients. In fact, a literature search reveals little information specific to addressing sexual health promotion within bachelor of science in nursing education programs. Sexual health has not been viewed as a priority in nursing care. Most programs include topics that focus on cultural competencies but do not specifically outline alternative gender or sexual identities as cultural perspectives that a new graduate may encounter. The papers that do focus on the sexual needs of individuals with chronic illnesses are targeted at advanced practitioners.

The AIDS epidemic triggered many to define sexual health and the urgent need to develop ways of promoting sexual health. Sexual health promotion is needed in many situations, however—not just those related to sexual infections; it is also an important issue in chronic illnesses, as demonstrated in the case study. This chapter begins by presenting operational definitions key to increasing the comfort levels of nurses relating to sexual health, discussing barriers nurses may encounter in addressing sexual health needs, and then outlining an assessment model that nurses can employ to help in their sexual health promotion practices.

Definitions

For one to live a fully healthy life, *sexual health* needs must be addressed. To deny the existence of sexuality is to limit the human experience. In Maslow's hierarchy of needs, sexuality is one of the basic needs, such as food, air, and water. When patients enter the healthcare setting, they do not become asexual. They might wear unisex gowns, but they do not have their sexuality locked up with their valuable possessions. Nursing assessments and interventions need to be thoughtful and careful, acknowledging the patient's right to privacy while providing the necessary care.

The term *sexual and reproductive health* for many may indicate specific topics, such as contraception and abortion, whereas *sexual health* includes a broad spectrum of topics. These topics include, but are not limited to, desire, condoms, emergency contraception, health care, sexuality and disability, sexual abuse, and sexuality in middle age and later life. The Sexuality Information and Education Council of the United States (SIECUS) was founded in 1964 to provide education and information about sexuality and sexual and reproductive health (http://www.siecus.org). Its website is a great resource for nurses for policy as well as teaching aids. SIECUS affirms that sexuality is a fundamental part of being human, one that is worthy of dignity, accurate information, comprehensive education about sexuality, and sexual health services. The World Health Organization's definition of sexual health includes the social aspects of this part of life: "Sexual health is a state of physical, mental and social wellbeing in relation to sexuality. It requires a positive and respectful approach to sexuality and sexual relationships, as well as the possibility of having pleasurable and safe sexual experiences, free of coercion, discrimination and violence."

Sex is physiologic, defined by one's male or female genitals. *Sexual orientation* is defined as the tendency to prefer romantic and sexual partners of the opposite sex, same sex, or both, or other; it is not a binary phenomenon. *Gender* is defined by one's psychological experience of one's sex. *Gender identity* is the subjective experience of being male or female. Gender identity develops early in childhood; to a large extent, it is a function of what one is taught and expected to do in a culture based on one's sex. *Gender roles* are all the behaviors that communicate the extent to which one is masculine/feminine/androgenous.

Barriers to Addressing Sexual Health Needs

There are several reasons why nurses may have difficulty discussing sexuality and sexual health with their patients. They may believe that they do not know enough to help their patients, they may be shy about the topic, they may fear that they will offend their patients, they may have no idea how to begin discussing the topic, or they may have conservative views about sexuality. Patients may also be shy about bringing up their concerns to health professionals and may be waiting for the health professional to bring up the topic.

Nurses can take several approaches to help overcome these potential barriers to communication. First and foremost, nurses need to reflect on their own beliefs and values related to sexuality and sexual health. Without this reflection, they can become prey to assumptions that will interfere with sexual health promotion. For example, heterosexism is a particular problem in our society. We make the assumption that someone is heterosexual and use language that can be offensive to our patients, such as "your wife/husband." It is best to use more neutral language, such as "your partner." We also have a tendency to think that older adults are asexual, even though we know that the ability to express sexuality remains important throughout the life span. Taking a self-sexual history includes reflecting on your own sexual education within your family, at school, and with friends. Completing this task will help you to be able to bracket your own issues so that you can work effectively with your clients.

Physical care for patients can sometimes lead to confusion about sexually appropriate behavior. Physical touch is a normal part of providing a great deal of nursing care; however, some patients could misunderstand it. When patients make sexually explicit remarks, engage in inappropriate touch, or make jokes that could be perceived as "off-color," some nurses may become uncomfortable and reluctant to spend time with the patient. Nurses should respond honestly and immediately to comments or touching that seems inappropriate. If this direct approach is ineffective, then nurses should discuss the matter with supervisors, social workers, and/or psychiatry departments to develop strategies for limiting patient behavior while providing the necessary care.

Nurses need to be aware that patients may misconstrue their behavior. Revealing clothes or talking about personal details of one's romantic life might confuse patients and blur the lines of the professional relationship between nurses and patients. It is important to remember that the focus of the nurse–patient relationship is always the patient. When a nurse is unsure if a conversation or behavior is appropriate, a trusted colleague may provide necessary feedback and suggest different approaches to working with the patient.

Sexual Health Assessment

Prior to beginning the sexual health assessment, some essential factors are critical to consider. Privacy is of utmost importance, so it will be key that you find a quiet, private area in which to talk. The more comfortable you are with the assessment, the more comfortable the client will be. Therefore role-playing an assessment/ management with a peer prior to an actual assessment will be very helpful in increasing your comfort level. The more sexual health assessments you complete, the easier they will become for you. When working with older adults, assessments should be performed in a respectful manner that conveys an understanding of the continuing sexual needs of older adults. The experience of illness and disability can change how patients express and maintain their sexuality. Nursing assessments and interventions need to be thoughtful and careful, acknowledging the patient's right to privacy while providing the necessary care.

The P-LI-SS-IT model is one of the most commonly used and effective models for assessment and intervention of sexual problems. Each stage will be defined here, and an example given.

The first step is "Permission," meaning giving the patient permission to have sexual feelings/relationships. It is also asking permission to discuss the patient's sexual health. For example, some women who have been diagnosed with breast cancer find that this disease affects their relationships and decreases their interest in sex. The nurse could tell her patient that this happens and ask her if she would like to discuss this issue.

The second step is "Limited Information," which means offering some information to identify the effect of the cancer/treatment on the patient's sexuality. This step is also a time to correct any misconceptions and provide accurate information. In this case, the woman may have mentioned to the nurse that the mastectomy has made her feel less attractive to her partner. The nurse could state, "You mentioned that you think you are less attractive to your partner. Have you talked to him about that?"

The third step is to provide "Specific Suggestions"—in this case, how to begin that conversation with her partner and maybe role-play starting a discussion so she feels comfortable opening the conversation with her partner. The fourth step is

"Intensive Therapy," where the nurse identifies the issues that need further support and refers her patient to the appropriate provider.

Summary

Becoming comfortable with completing a sexual health assessment and caring for the sexual health needs of our patients can be challenging. Nurses need not feel that they have to be prepared to help their patients through the four steps of the P-LI-SS-IT model. In fact, as a nurse without further training in sexuality education, even helping patients through the first few steps of this model would be a wonderful help to the patients. Furthermore, the major tasks for a nurse are to examine his or her own beliefs and values about sexuality and to be willing to be open in a nonjudgmental way to the many ways people express their sexuality.

Case Study Resolution

For L.S. and W.N., as newlyweds, the nurses need to help them be open to exploring different positions that would accommodate both her limited range of motion and his shortness of breath. It is not so important that the nurse feels competent in suggesting the actual positions, but rather simply that he or she is open to suggesting that the couple think about positioning as an option. The couple will probably be able to work it out themselves with the suggestion. Because the nurse was open with them, they will probably be comfortable discussing their sexual needs with the nurse if problems continue, which would allow the nurse to make a referral to a specialist as needed.

EXERCISES

1. Individually answer the following questions and reflect on your answers:

   a. How often, when you were young, did you see your parent(s) in the nude? What was your family's attitude toward nudity?

   b. If you ever have children, do you hope to be more accepting of nudity in your family than your parent(s), less accepting, or about the same?

   c. How did you first learn about or discover masturbation, and how did you feel about it at first?

    d. If you masturbated when you were younger, did you ever let anyone else know about it?

    e. If you masturbate now, how do you feel about the practice? Are you guilty? Ashamed? Happy? Proud? Disgusted? Satisfied?

    f. Make a list of the sex-related slang terms that you feel comfortable using, if any (e.g., "screwing," "fuck," "cock").

    g. Which of the words on the list would your parents have been comfortable using?

    h. Which of the words on the list would be offensive to you if you heard them being spoken by a friend of the other gender? Of the same gender?

2. Read the following case and as a group work through the questions.

Mr. B. is a 45-year-old construction worker who was admitted to the emergency room (ER) following a serious fall at work. The ER team begins to undress him to assess the full extent of his injuries. When they remove his outer work clothing, they find he is wearing female underclothes.

    a. What is your reaction when faced with an embarrassing situation? Using the P-LI-SS-IT model, can you identify the level at which you would be able to work with Mr. B.?

    b. Because of the short-term nature of emergency care, how easy or difficult is it for staff to deal with a patient's sexuality and sexual health?

    c. People who cross-dress vary in their sexual orientation. How would you promote nonprejudicial care for Mr. B.?

Additional Resources

Albaugh, J. A., & Kellogg-Spadt, K. (2003). Sexuality and the nurse's role and initial approach to patients. *Urologic Nursing, 23*, 227–228.

Annon, J. S. (1976). The PLISSIT model: A proposed conceptual scheme for the behavioral treatment of sexual problems. *Journal of Sex Education Therapists, 2*, 1–15.

Ayaz, S., & Kubilay, G. (2009). Effectiveness of the PLISSIT model for solving the sexual problems of patients with stoma. *Journal of Clinical Nursing, 18*, 89–98.

Brown, A. P., Lubman, D. I., & Paxton, S. J (2008). STIs and blood borne viruses: Risk factors for individuals with mental illness. *Australian Family Physician, 37*, 531–534.

Burrows, G. (2011). Lesbian, gay, bisexual and transgender health. Part 1: Sexual orientation. *Practice Nurse, 41*, 23–25.

Dahir, M. (2011). A sexual medicine health care model and nurse practitioner role. *Urologic Nursing, 31*, 359–362.

Irwin, R. (1997). Sexual health promotion and nursing. *Journal of Advanced Nursing, 25*, 170–177.

Nicolaou, L. (2011). Sexual dysfunction in people with schizophrenia. *Mental Health Practice, 15*, 20–24.

Ouzts, K. N., Brown, J. W., & Swearingen, C. A. D. (2006). Developing public health competence among RN-to-BSN students in a rural community. *Public Health Nursing, 23*, 178–182.

Quinn, C., & Browne, G. (2009). Sexuality of people living with mental illness: A collaborative challenge for mental health nurses. *International Journal of Mental Health Nursing, 18*, 195–203.

Royal College of Nursing. (2000). *Sexuality and sexual health in nursing practice.* RCN Publication Code 0009650. London, UK: Author.

World Health Organization. (1987). *Concepts of sexual health. Report of a working group convened by the World Health Organization (EURO).* Copenhagen, Denmark: Author.

World Health Organization. (2011). Sexual health. Retrieved from http://www.who.int/topics/sexual_health/en

CHAPTER FOURTEEN

Helping Patients with Pain

Jeannine Brant, PhD, APRN, AOCN

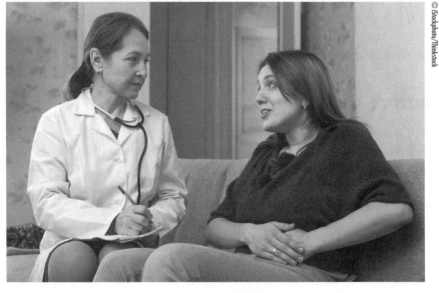

© iStockphoto/Thinkstock

■ CASE STUDY

Marianne is a 73-year-old woman who reported being in good health until approximately 2 months ago. She was working in her garden and began to experience low back and neck pain. She treated her pain with rest, warm rice bags, and acetaminophen. Unfortunately, her pain persisted, and Marianne sought medical attention. Magnetic resonance imaging (MRI) revealed abnormal changes in her cervical and lumbar spine. A follow-up bone scan suggested malignancy, and her complete blood count revealed that she was anemic. A bone marrow biopsy followed, and Marianne was diagnosed with multiple myeloma. Due to the instability of her cervical spine, she was hospitalized and placed in a soft collar, and radiation therapy was promptly initiated.

During the change of shift report, the nurse reported that the patient denied pain and required no pain medication. Pain scores were documented over the past 2 days since admission as 0 on a 0–10 scale, with 0 being "no pain" and 10 being the "worst possible pain." The clinical nurse specialist (CNS), who was familiar with the pain normally associated with multiple myeloma, questioned the pain scores and decided to further assess the patient. Upon entering the room, the CNS noticed that the patient was lying on her back with the head of the bed slightly elevated and the cervical collar was in place. When the CNS asked Marianne to rate her pain, she stated, "0." The CNS further questioned the patient about pain with movement, and the patient replied, "I don't move. I just lie still, because it hurts too much when I move." Clearly, the lack of communication with the patient interfered with her pain control, mobility, and quality of life.

Introduction

Pain is a significant problem in patients throughout the life cycle and is a major reason why patients seek health care. All individuals will experience pain at some point during their life. It is estimated that as many as 80% of patients who are hospitalized experience pain, and approximately 53% of patients with cancer experience pain sometime during the disease process. In the United States, chronic pain burdens approximately 100 million adults. According to the Institute of Medicine (IOM, 2011), pain constitutes a crisis, and a multitude of barriers exist related to its assessment and management. Pain not only has physical consequences but also affects healing, functional status, psychological and social well-being, hospital length of stay, and healthcare costs.

It is a nursing-sensitive indicator, so nurses play a key role in successful pain management. Nurses must learn how to effectively communicate with patients to adequately assess and manage pain while at the same time recognizing barriers that interfere with optimal care.

Assessment of Pain

Communication about pain begins with the pain assessment. Nurses should learn how to adequately and comprehensively assess pain using a systematic approach. They should also be aware of the barriers that can interfere with the pain assessment.

Pain Assessment

Pain is a subjective experience that can only be defined by the individual. Pain is defined as "whatever the experiencing person says it is existing whenever he or she says it does" (McCaffery, 1968). Because pain is a subjective phenomenon, nurses need to communicate with patients about the presence and experience of pain. As indicated in the case study, nurses often need communication strategies that reveal the true story of each person's pain. The acronym OLDCART can serve as a reminder of the important questions for pain assessment:

- **O**: Onset of the pain
- **L**: Location(s)
- **D**: Duration—how long the patient has been experiencing the pain
- **C**: Characteristics—pain intensity, pain with movement, words used to describe the pain
- **A**: Aggravating factors—what makes the pain worse
- **R**: Relieving factors—what makes the pain better
- **T**: Treatment—which treatments have been tried and which ones work

Once this information is gathered, the assessment can be used to inform other healthcare team members of the patient's experience (Brant, 2012).

The patient's personal pain goal (0–10 pain score defined by the patient) should be also be obtained during the assessment.

Communication techniques may vary between groups. For example, older adults understand and communicate differently than young children. Some patients may be nonverbal, preverbal, or unable to verbally communicate their pain experience (Herr, Bjoro, & Decker, 2006). Table 14-1 includes tips on communicating with different populations.

Assessment Barriers

Patient-related and healthcare team barriers to communication can impede a complete pain assessment. Patients may deny pain due to their perception of pain as a weakness, fears that their disease is progressing, or even the belief that pain is an inevitable part of illness or aging. A patient may want to be a "good patient"

Table 14-1 Pain Assessment in Different Populations

Population	Comments
Older adults	• Try to obtain a self-report, even in patients with dementia.
	• Speak clearly and loud enough to be heard.
	• Patients may prefer a vertical thermometer to rate pain over a horizontal one.
Nonverbal adults	• Use a five-step approach:
	1. Try to obtain a self-report of pain.
	2. Look for indicators that pain is likely to be present (e.g., trauma, disease).
	3. Use a nonverbal behavioral scale to assess the pain (e.g., Checklist of Nonverbal Pain Indicators).
	4. Obtain a surrogate report, as a loved one who knows the patient may inform the assessment about the possible presence of pain.
	5. Try an analgesic trial to see if pain behaviors subside.
Children	• Try to obtain a self-report—even young children can report pain.
	• Use a Faces rating scale.
	• Use a tool for preverbal children (e.g., Face–Legs–Activity–Cry–Consolability [FLACC]).

and not bother the nurse or team with complaints of pain. Some patients fear addiction to pain medications or the side effects associated with analgesics. When a patient appears to be in more pain than reported, or when the pain assessment is not consistent with the disease process (as in the case study), a more thorough assessment may be indicated to further explore the individual's pain perceptions.

For healthcare teams, attitudes and beliefs about pain can interfere with the pain assessment. Often, these beliefs are displayed with nonverbal behaviors such as grimacing. A compassionate, nonjudgmental attitude from the nurse is essential in establishing a trust relationship with the patient. This attitude is important regardless of whether the patient's report of pain is believable. The nurse can validate the patient's report of pain and then deliver strategies to control unrelieved pain as indicated. Patients often have fears about addiction that are unfounded and may interfere with good pain management. When addiction to pain medications is suspected, that concern should be communicated with the physician and other healthcare team members.

Management of Pain

Pain management involves a multimodal approach that includes both pharmacologic and nonpharmacologic strategies (American Pain Society, 2008). Often, multiple strategies are needed to provide optimal pain management. These strategies may overwhelm patients and families. The nurse plays an integral role in communicating the pain management care plan to the patient and family to lessen this perceived burden of information.

Patient Education

Because pharmacologic treatments are the mainstay of pain management, sufficient time should be spent teaching patients and their caregivers about the prescribed medications. The nurse should discuss the rationale for each medication, the schedule and instructions for administration, antici-pated side effects, and when to call the prescribing clinician (Table 14-2) (Joint Commission, 2012). Often, medications such as antidepressants and anticonvulsants are also ordered to manage pain, but patients may be confused about the role of these medicines in the pain management. If this information is not explained, patients may feel that the healthcare team is not being truthful. For example, the patient may perceive that the doctor believes he or she is depressed

Table 14-2 Communicating About Pain Medications

Communication Message	Comments
Reason for the medication	• Several medications may be ordered for pain. • Patients may lack understanding that each medication works in a unique way.
How often to take the medication	• Confusion often exists about long-acting versus breakthrough pain medications. • Instruct patients about when to begin a new medication, especially if there is a delay.
Administration instructions	• Specific instructions should indicate if the medication needs to be taken with food or on an empty stomach. • Food and drug interactions should be acknowledged.
Side effects of the medication	• Uncontrolled side effects can lead to nonadherence or safety concerns. • Constipation is a universal side effect of opioids; patients should understand the need to take a prophylactic stool softener and bowel stimulant. • Opioids can cause sedation and lead to falls; patients should be instructed not to drive if sedation occurs.

When to call the doctor	• Patients should call for:
	  • Inadequate relief of pain
	  • Uncontrolled side effects of the pain medications
	  • Questions about the pain management plan of care

and, therefore, ordered an antidepressant without the patient's knowledge. Long-acting (LA) and breakthrough medications may involve the same opioid (e.g., morphine) and can lead to confusion about proper administration. Patients should understand that the LA medications should be taken around the clock

Figure 14-1   Illustration of the Effects of Long-Acting and Breakthrough Analgesics

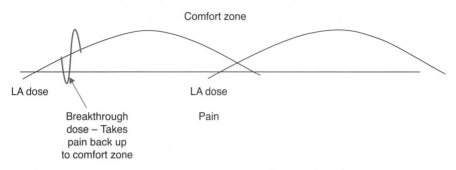

and that breakthrough medications should be taken on an *as needed* basis. Using analogies, such as the LA medication being *sprinkled* into the system over time, can help with understanding. Drawing a diagram that highlights the differences between LA and breakthrough medications is also helpful for some patients (Figure 14-1).

Medication List and Reconciliation

The list of pain medications should be reconciled at every visit (i.e., listed by name, dosage, and schedule). This list should include the addition of new medications, discontinuation of previous medications, and specific transitions in care such as hospital discharge or change to hospice care. This list serves as an important communication link between healthcare providers and settings. In addition, patients may become confused about which medications they should continue and which ones should be permanently discontinued, so reconciliation is also an assessment of patient self-care strategies and understanding. Unused medication should be disposed of properly to prevent inadvertent administration or diversion. Written instructions with a reconciled list of medications should be given the patient at each transition in care.

Nonpharmacologic Management

Nonpharmacologic modalities are often used to manage or augment other pain management strategies. These treatments include ice, heat, massage, splinting, relaxation, distraction, and other options. Nurses should suggest the addition of these strategies and provide clear instructions about their safety and appropriate use. For example, heat may not be appropriate for patients with diabetes or neuropathy. Nonpharmacologic therapies are an important and cost-effective approach to pain management.

Healthcare Team Communication

Managing pain is not an easy task. Once the pain is assessed, the nurse and healthcare team need to decide on appropriate interventions to provide comfort. The team presents these interventions so patients have an opportunity to decide on the management strategies and goals of treatment. After implementation of the selected interventions, nurses reassess patients for the effectiveness and side effects of the interventions. When interventions are not effective, the nurse plays a primary role in communicating the lack of efficacy to the prescribing clinician and healthcare team and then suggesting alternative strategies that may be more effective or tolerable. Nurses also advocate for pain assessment and management at shift reports, during rounds in the hospital, and at team meetings to facilitate communication and success of the pain management plan.

Summary

- Patient satisfaction scores reflect the adequacy of communication between the nurse and the patient.
- A formal pain management plan should be communicated to each patient.
- Communication about pain improves patient satisfaction with care.
- Nurses have opportunities to make changes in pain outcomes, and communication about pain is a key strategy in every quality improvement effort.

Case Study Resolution

After obtaining a more comprehensive pain assessment from Marianne, the nurse calls the physician to discuss the assessment findings. She reports that Marianne's pain is a 0 at rest but a 9 with movement and activity. Because the pain is so severe with any type of movement, the patient is started on long-acting morphine sulfate, along with intravenous patient-controlled analgesia (PCA) for the breakthrough pain. The nurse discusses the use of the PCA and encourages Marianne to self-administer a dose of morphine prior to activities that cause pain, such as getting out of bed, turning over in bed, and eating. The nurse also reinforces the need for good pain control to facilitate healing, movement, and overall quality of life. Within 24 hours, Marianne's pain is well controlled, with pain reported as being a 4 with movement. She is able to sit in the chair and move around her room with a pain level that matches her pain goal.

Websites

American Pain Society

The American Pain Society is a multidisciplinary community that brings together a diverse group of scientists, clinicians, and other professionals to increase the knowledge of pain and transform public policy and clinical practice to reduce pain-related suffering. Clinical practice guidelines and patient education materials are available.

http://www.ampainsoc.org/about/

City of Hope Pain and Palliative Care Center (COHPPRC)

COHPPRC is a central source that collects a variety of materials, including pain assessment tools and patient education materials.

http://prc.coh.org

End of Life/Palliative Education Resource Center (EPERC), Medical College of Wisconsin

The purpose of EPERC is to share educational resource materials among the community of health professional educators involved in palliative care education. It provides several educational examples relevant to pain assessment and management.

http://www.eperc.mcw.edu/EPERC/FastFactsIndex

Joint Commission Resources

Joint Commission Resources (JCR) is dedicated to helping healthcare organizations prosper by improving quality of care and patient safety, and managing pain is a high priority for JCR.

http://www.jcrinc.com/APM10/Extras/

The Resource Center (TRC) for the Alliance of State Pain Initiatives

TRC provides excellent tools to support organizational change and professional education to improve pain management.

http://trc.wisc.edu/index.asp

Evidence-Based Article

Martin, L., Kelly, M. J., & Roosa, K. (2012). Multidisciplinary approach to improving pain management. *Critical Care Nursing Quarterly, 35*, 268–271.

Improving pain management is a complex and challenging endeavor. This article describes the pain care challenges on a 30-bed trauma surgical unit and reports pain improvement efforts that led to successful strategies to improve pain care. The Hospital Consumer Assessment of Health Providers and Systems (HCAHPS) survey was used to monitor success of the pain improvement efforts. Initially, the unit was in the 68th percentile for the HCAHPS pain score, far below an acceptable level. Patients were also expressing dissatisfaction with their pain care, especially in regard to wound care. A best practice group was convened to brainstorm possible factors that were contributing to pain care dissatisfaction. Pain plan communication was listed as a major gap in care. To address this gap, nurses developed a teaching tool that involved communication of the pain care plan to the patient. Pain during wound care was also discussed, and nurses met with trauma surgeons to identify a solution for better pain control. Other efforts arose from these meetings, and the team eventually addressed the pain experience during the entire surgical patient's stay. The unit moved to the 90th percentile in HCAHPS scores following implementation of the efforts.

References

American Pain Society. (2008). *Principles of analgesic use in the treatment of acute pain and cancer pain* (6th ed.). Glenview, IL: APS Press.

Brant, J. M. (2012). Strategies to manage pain in palliative care. In M. O'Connor, S. Lee, & S. Aranda (Eds.), *Palliative care nursing: A guide to practice* (3rd ed., pp. 93–113). Victoria, Australia: Ausmed.

Herr, K., Bjoro, K., & Decker, S. (2006). Tools for assessment of pain in nonverbal older adults with dementia: A state-of-the-science review. *Journal of Pain Symptom Management, 31*(2), 170–192.

Institute of Medicine. (2011). *Relieving pain in America*. Washington, DC: Author.

Joint Commission (Ed.). (2012). *Approaches to pain management: An essential guide for clinical leaders*. Oak Brook, IL: Author.

McCaffery, M. (1968). *Nursing practice: Theories related to cognition, bodily pain, and man–environment interactions*. Los Angeles, CA: UCLA Student Store.

CHAPTER FIFTEEN

Communication in Life-Threatening Illness and Spiritual Care

Amy Rex-Smith

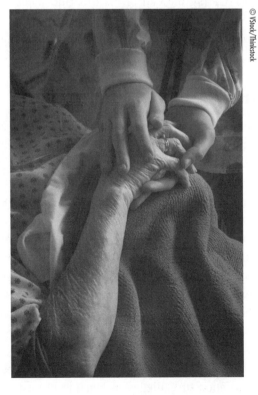

■ CASE STUDY

Mr. T., who likes to be known as Mike, is a 57-year-old man with multiple myeloma. For the past 7 years, he has tried every possible treatment for his disease, from steroids and thalidomide to a bone marrow transplant. During his illness, he returned to the Episcopal faith of his childhood. He has been attending weekly healing services at the local parish, where the priest has been praying for Mike's healing from cancer with the "laying on of hands" on Mike's head as he kneels at the altar. In addition, several months ago Mike reconciled with his brother, with whom he had not spoken since their mother's death 8 years earlier.

Today Mike arrives in the outpatient unit with shortness of breath, confusion, and a blood pressure of 58/38 mm Hg. Mike is still talking and is very clear that he does not want to be resuscitated. The team is prepared to order "comfort measures only" (CMO) and to initiate a hospice referral. His wife knows that Mike is nearing the end of his life. She states, "I don't know what to expect.... I want him to be comfortable, but I just can't understand why God hasn't healed Mike, when he has been so faithful in attending the prayer service every week."

Introduction

For patients and their families, the diagnosis of an illness that may be life shortening is a frightening prospect. In such a scenario, the expected togetherness of shared events and family milestones becomes clouded by the shadow of loss. For many patients, this type of illness represents an existential crisis, which raises concerns about their spirituality. For these patients, their spiritual needs can become a primary focus.

Nursing interventions can have a significant impact on the patient's adjustment to a changed vision of the future. Nurses work in many different settings where patients deal with life-altering illnesses—from nurses who care for patients before cardiac bypass surgery to hospice nurses who help patients with terminal cancer reach their end-of-life goals. Nurses can make the process of facing life-threatening illness more bearable and even enriching for patients and their families. In addition, addressing spiritual concerns is expected when giving end-of-life care (Ferrell, LaPorte Matzo, Penn, Sheehan, & Sherman, 2003). The American Association of Colleges of Nursing has established standardized national education for nurses in end-of-life care, which are available for further reference (http://www.aacn.nche.edu/elnec).

Life-Threatening Illness

In a culture that fears death, the specter of dying can be overwhelming to the patient with a life-threatening diagnosis. The patient may experience emotional and spiritual distress related to the potential changes in his or her functioning and shortened life expectancy. The disease process and treatments can affect the physical, psychosocial, spiritual, and financial aspects of a patient's and his or her family's life. Patients may experience anticipatory grieving regarding future losses and unfinished life business. Nurses are in a unique position to help patients and their families adjust to and cope with changes due to an illness and its treatment, find support from multiple sources including their faith tradition and their loved ones, and discover meaning in their lives and impending death (Box 15-1).

In her landmark work, Elizabeth Kübler-Ross (1969) described the stages of death and dying: denial, anger, bargaining, depression, and acceptance. Today these same stages are also used to describe the process of grieving and even the acceptance of a diagnosis of life-threatening illness. While each patient is unique, nurses can use these stages as a framework for understanding the variety of responses that patients may demonstrate while trying to cope with a potentially shortened life span. These are not sequential stages but rather a way to understand and then explain to patients what may be normal responses during a stressful time.

Nurses are in a unique position to help patients and their families prepare for change brought on by illness.

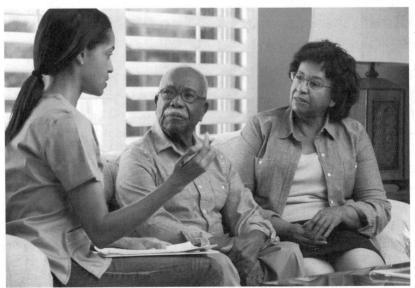

© Monkey Business Images/ShutterStock, Inc.

Box 15-1 Talking with Patients About Life-Threatening Illness

---

- Explain the disease and treatment, using other healthcare providers to deliver information and answer questions that are not within the realm of nursing. For example, the physician can discuss the prognosis or the results of diagnostic tests.

- Allow ample time for the patient to discuss his or her thoughts, feelings, and fears about the diagnosis and treatment and their impact on his or her life.

- Help the patient explore sources of support and previous methods of coping that have been successful (e.g., talking with significant others, reading about the illness or searching the Internet for related sites, talking with clergy, joining a support group, meditating).

- Work with the patient and family when making decisions about care to enhance their sense of control over what may be a frightening situation.

- Observe the patient for signs of ineffective coping patterns and/or psychiatric disorders (anxiety, depression, suicidal ideas) that require further assessment, intervention, or referral.

- Provide positive feedback for the patient's use of coping strategies that work.

- Address the patient's concerns about symptom control: pain relief and control of nausea, with possible interventions if problems arise.

- Suggest other sources of information and support including support groups, websites, and community organizations.

Spiritual Assessment: Meeting Standards for Patient-Centered Care

Spiritual assessment is a required element of nursing assessment and is essential for providing comprehensive nursing care. Because spirituality and religion are regarded as personal areas that are not addressed in everyday social interactions, beginning nurses may be reluctant to address these concerns with their patients. However, because healthcare decisions are often based on these personal beliefs, spirituality and religion can affect critical aspects of patient health. Thus spiritual care is an accepted part of nursing practice.

The ability to become proficient in spiritual care starts with the knowledge of how to do a spiritual assessment and improves with experience. While every nurse will not become an expert in spiritual care, every nurse is required to meet the Quality and Safety Education for Nurses (QSEN, 2007) criteria (http://qsen.org/) of providing safe, high-quality, patient-centered care. To meet this standard, a religious and spiritual assessment is required. Identification of a patient's spiritual needs often makes the difference between clinical care that is individualized and meaningful to the patient and excellent physical care that misses the spiritual mark. This is especially true in end-of-life situations.

Spiritual assessment is not a one-time event, but rather is ongoing, as the patient's spiritual needs may change as a result of the illness experience and disease progression (McSherry & Ross, 2011). Spiritual assessment covers three topics: general spiritual status, spiritual needs, and spiritual resources. A screening spiritual assessment can be kept very simple, by asking questions such as "Is your faith important in your life?" and "How does your faith affect your health care?" Many spiritual assessment tools have been developed for general use and for specific patient settings. For example, for patients who are hospitalized, screening questions such as "Are there any religious or spiritual practices that would be helpful to you while you are here?" and "Would you like to see a chaplain?" are sufficient. For a sampling of spiritual assessment tools, see the web resources at the end of this chapter.

Guidelines for Spiritual Care Interventions

Some spiritual care interventions are within the nurse's scope of practice. These include creating space and time for religious rituals, providing support by making connections to the patient's faith community or clergy/spiritual advisors, and making referrals to chaplaincy (Rex Smith, 2006). In addition, attentive listening and "presence" (communicating caring without using words) are accepted nursing interventions, each of which is described in detail in the next two sections. Praying with patients at their request has also entered the mainstream of accepted interventions, although not every nurse may be comfortable with offering a verbal prayer. Nurses should not offer spiritual advice unless they have received specialized training. Table 15-1 provides helpful communication guidelines for spiritual care that were developed by Dr. Harold G. Koenig (2008) at the Duke Center for Spirituality, Theology and Health (http://www.spiritualityandhealth.duke.edu).

Table 15-1 Dr. Koenig's Guidelines for Spiritual Care Interventions

Dr. Koenig's Do's	Dr. Koenig's Don'ts
Do take a spiritual history.	*Don't* continue taking a spiritual history if the patient is not religious and indicates discomfort or resistance to such questioning.
Do support the patient's beliefs.	*Don't* prescribe religion to nonreligious patients or proselytize.
Do say a short prayer if requested by the patient (if you are able/comfortable with prayer).	*Don't* pray with a patient without a previous spiritual history and pray only if the patient asks.
Do refer spiritual needs to chaplains and develop relationships with local chaplains and clergy.	*Don't* provide spiritual counsel or advice (unless you have had specialized training in spiritual care).
Do alter the healthcare environment to accommodate religious rituals and practices.	*Don't* argue with patients about their religious beliefs, even when those beliefs conflict with medical or nursing care.

Source: Adapted from Koenig, H. G. (2008). Clinical applications. In *Medicine, religion and health*. West Conshohocken, PA: Templeton Press. Used with permission.

Attentive Listening

Nurses who practice attentive listening are attuned to the ordinary cues routinely offered by patients that may indicate their spiritual and emotional needs or suggest how they are coping with illness. Nurses caring for this special population must be alert to listen for issues in the spiritual realm. Patients may or may not be overtly religious or follow a specific faith tradition, yet they may express issues concerning spirituality during conversations. Nurses can learn to identify cues that indicate spiritual needs. Nurses should be willing and able to provide support during the patient's journey throughout the illness. According to Carson and Koenig (2004), the following four spiritual issues are apt to arise when facing life-threatening illness:

1. Needs for forgiveness and reconciliation
2. Needs for prayer and religious services
3. Spiritual assistance at death
4. A sense of peace

Presence: Communicating Caring Without Using Words

Presence is a specialized nursing intervention. The goal of presence is patient well-being. The essential feature for presence to occur is that the nurse must be physically present with the patient, focused on the patient, and completely available to the patient. Both inner and outer distractions will prevent presence from being able to occur. Presence is often experienced by patients when a nurse sits quietly at the bedside. This often occurs after a nurse–patient conversation has ended, as the nurse and patient let companionable silence emerge between them. The nurse is fully attentive to the patient. Speech is not required; silence is the norm. The nurse enters the patient's personal space and maintains a focus on the patient and his or her environment. The nurse seeks to have an openness to the entire situation. A sense of transcendence—that is, connectedness to something outside of oneself—may or may not occur when presence is utilized. Nurses who experience transcendence routinely as part of their personal faith tradition practices may be more likely to have this experience with patients in the clinical setting (Rex Smith, 2007).

Advance Directives

Communication between patients and their healthcare providers is enhanced by advance directives. *Advance directives* is an umbrella term for several documents that explain the patient's wishes for cardiopulmonary resuscitation, tube feedings, and advanced life support in addition to designating other people who may make healthcare decisions if the patient is unable to do so. These documents may include a living will, a durable power of attorney, a healthcare proxy, and advance medical directives. Regulations regarding each of these documents vary by state and country. If the patient becomes unable to participate in decisions about his or her care, advance directives provide the legal guidelines for healthcare interventions.

Ideally, discussion about advance directives should occur between patients and their primary healthcare providers in a non-acute situation when the patient is able to participate and express his or her wishes. In contrast, in an acute crisis, anxiety, medications, level of consciousness, or pain may cloud the decision-making process. Patients should also be encouraged to include and share their wishes with their families or identified healthcare proxy. Advance directives are an important means of relaying patients' end-of-life goals when they are no longer able or competent to make their wishes known.

Palliative Care: More Than End-of-Life Care

Palliative care focuses on quality of life by providing adequate symptom control and promoting comfort (Campbell, 2008). Many providers have confounded hospice care with palliative care. Palliative care focuses on symptom management and may begin at any time; hospice care is usually defined as care for the last 6 months of life. Palliative care may be instituted at any time after a patient receives a diagnosis, although it is still most often associated with end-of-life care. Palliative care is often initiated when the disease progresses and causes more problematic symptoms. Care during a life-shortening illness builds upon the physical care that provides adequate treatment and comfort. Physical care is essential, as symptoms that are not well controlled may cause physical discomfort and prevent the patient from addressing psychosocial, emotional, and spiritual needs. While there are many acronyms to describe the goals of palliative care, two commonly used terms are *comfort measures only* (CMO) and *allow natural death* (AND) (Campbell, 2008).

Even with adequate advance care directives, the patient and family may become bewildered by the array of options and may seek permission to focus on comfort care and grieving. Often members of the healthcare team may offer information that is conflicting, and the situation can get confusing for patients and their families. Family meetings with the entire healthcare team are often needed to be able to clarify care goals. This is not an event but a process: Ongoing clarification of the patient's wishes and goals is critical, given that treatment decisions change as the patient's condition changes. While the focus of palliative care is improved quality of life, recent studies have explored the value of earlier initiation of palliative care in specific patient populations, with some initial evidence suggesting that earlier institution of palliative care may also extend the length of life (Jacobsen et al., 2011).

Grief, Loss, and Mourning

The impending or actual loss of a loved one can be an overwhelming event for the patient's family and friends. For example, suppose a 56-year-old woman dies in the emergency room after a cardiac arrest. The family is in the waiting room. After the emergency room physician tells the family about her death, the nurse is in a unique position to listen and console the family during the initial shock and grieving. The nurse's education in communication and the grief process provides useful strategies when intervening with those experiencing loss (Box 15-2). Experienced nurses provide specific interventions to help family and friends, such as identifying coping skills and support mechanisms, helping family members manage, and connecting them to available resources during times of crisis.

As the patient nears the end of life and is kept comfortable, the focus of nursing care often shifts to the patient's family. Family members may also experience health problems during the grief process, leading them to seek health care. Common physical symptoms during grieving are loss of appetite, sleeplessness, shortness of breath, tightness in the neck, a feeling of hollowness or tightness in the chest, lack of energy, dry mouth, and muscle weakness. Grieving is a universal emotion; in addition to feelings of sadness, grieving people may feel isolated, angry, guilty, lonely, numb, or helpless. They might cry, sigh, and be unable to concentrate. The process of grieving has many different patterns, and unless the symptoms are overly intense or persist for a long period of time, they are normal reactions to the loss of a loved one.

The prospect of limited time is frightening for patients and families.

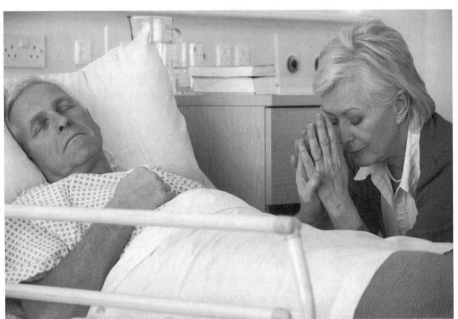

© Monkey Business Images/ShutterStock, Inc.

Box 15-2 Communicating with Grieving People

- Listen to the person's experience, helping the survivor to express his or her feelings.
- Assess the grieving person's support systems: family, friend, clergy, or confidantes with whom the person can talk freely.
- Be present and actively listen to the person's experience of grief.
- Allow ample time for the person to repeat the story of the death.
- Encourage discussion about what the future might be like without the deceased, what they will miss, what new roles the survivors will take on, etc.
- Avoid the use of rote responses like, "You'll be better in no time," "It was his time," or "She's better off now."
- Allow for individual differences in grieving because sometimes people "hear the voice" of a loved one or "miss their smell."
- Suggest support groups that help family members and children who have experienced the loss of a loved one.
- Refer people with prolonged grieving, depression, or suicidal ideas to an appropriate counselor.

Nurses can help those who are grieving the loss of a loved one. Mourning is the way of dealing with the grieving process within cultural and religious traditions, and each family member may experience it differently. Bowlby (1980) provides a helpful framework that describes four stages of mourning: (1) Phase of numbness: General feeling of numbness and possibly denial; (2) Phase of yearning and searching: Trying to find loved one but cannot, possibly feel or smell them, reality starts to set in; (3) Phase of disorganization and despair: Giving up hope of finding loved one, feeling hopeless, apathetic, depressed; and (4) Phase of reorganization: Seeking to remake life, establish new relationships. Effective nursing interventions include listening to family members' feelings and memories, identifying support systems that are available to them, helping them to verbalize how the loss has changed their world and expectations, and celebrating the positive lessons and stories that are part of their shared history.

While grieving is often described in stages, the actual process is individual and unique and may not proceed in an orderly fashion. Worden (1991) proposed four tasks of mourning. *Tasks* implies the "work" of grieving for the lost loved one and the acknowledgment that such work requires time, emotional effort, and concentration. The four tasks of mourning as described by Worden follow:

1. Accept the reality of the loss.
2. Work through the pain of grief.
3. Adjust to the environment in which the deceased is missing.
4. Relocate the deceased emotionally and move on with life.

There is a wide range of what is a normal length of time for mourning; it may take many years for a person to deal with a loss. Therefore, nurses need to be attentive to symptoms of prolonged grieving that interfere with normal life activities, such as work and family roles, or to thoughts or plans for suicide. These symptoms, especially thoughts of suicide, indicate the need for referral to other healthcare providers.

Summary

The diagnosis of a potentially life-shortening illness is a frightening prospect for patients and their families. This is a time when spiritual concerns often become more pressing. Adequate patient-centered care includes spiritual assessment for all patients and provision of individualized spiritual care based on the assessment findings. Nursing interventions such as attentive listening and presence can have a significant impact on patients' adjustment to a changed vision of their future. Nurses are in a unique position to help patients and their families cope with illness and treatment, find support in their loved ones, and discover meaning in life and death. Nurses can facilitate the process of coping and make loss more bearable and even a time of personal growth and connectedness for patients and their families. Appropriate spiritual care and interventions for anticipatory grieving lay the foundation for helping families move through the mourning process. Nursing interventions may be able to help family members come to terms with the loss of their loved one and help them avoid chronic grief and destructive reactions to the loss.

Case Study Resolution

The nurse recognized that the wife's concern was a cue that an immediate spiritual assessment was required. The nurse recognized that the answer to the theological question about God was beyond her purview, so she sat with the patient and wife, listened attentively, and offered her presence, as she sought to understand and clarify their concerns. She then collaborated with the physician, who visited with Mike and his family to discuss the actual physical aspects of dying and the potential amount of time left. The physician also explained the meaning of CMO and the referral to hospice. Because of the nurse's concern about the wife's expectation of healing from cancer, the nurse asked if she could make a referral to the hospice chaplain. With the permission of the patient and his wife, the nurse made the chaplaincy referral and explained that the wife had expected healing from the cancer. She also explained that the local Episcopal priest had been providing the spiritual care. The chaplain knew the priest well and had worked with her often; he was able to ensure that the patient's own priest and faith community would be available to provide support and spiritual care during the hospice home care.

Mike's wife was also worried about Mike falling in the shower. The nurse said, "Home care and hospice services could help with daily physical care and help you, as a family, during this time." Mike's two daughters, who lived nearby, visited daily and were a great source of help and support. Mike's brother was also able to visit, and Mike and his brother had a time of reminiscence and sibling connection that Mike relished. Mike often talked about how important the forgiveness of and reconciliation with his brother was to him.

Mike eventually slipped into a coma. Two days later, Mike died in his home, quietly, with his wife and daughters and his priest by his side.

Websites

Tools for Spiritual Assessment

Faith, Importance, Community, Address (FICA) (Puchalski, 2000)
   http://www.hpsm.org/documents/End_of_Life_Summit_FICA_References.pdf
   Spirituality and Medical Practice: Using the HOPE Questions as a Practical Tool for Spiritual Assessment
   Hope, Organized, Personal, Effects (HOPE) (Anandarajah & Hight, 2001)
   http://www.aafp.org/afp/2001/0101/p81.html

Resources for Palliative Care

   http://www.aacn.nche.edu/elnec
   http://www.nationalconsensusproject.org/

Oncology Nursing Society Spiritual Care Toolkit
http://www.new.towson.edu/sct/mandate.htm
Duke Center for Theology, Spirituality and Health
http://www.spiritualityandhealth.duke.edu

Evidence-Based Article

Maciejewski, P. K., Phelps, A. C., Kacel, E. L., Balboni, T. A., Balboni, M., Wright, A. A., ... Prigerson, H. G. (2012). Religious coping and behavioral disengagement: Opposing influences on advance care planning and receipt of intensive care near death. *Psycho-Oncology, 21*(7), 714–723. doi:10.1002/pon.1967

The researchers wanted to determine the relationships between methods of coping with advanced cancer, completion of advance care directives, and receipt of intensive, life-prolonging care near death. A total of 345 patients with advanced cancer were interviewed and then followed until they died. Contrary to what had been expected, positive religious coping was associated with lower rates of having a living will (adjusted odds ratio [AOR] = 0.39, $p = 0.003$) and predicted higher rates of intensive, life-prolonging care near death (AOR, 5.43; $p < 0.001$). Behavioral disengagement (giving up on trying to cope) was associated with higher rates of do-not-resuscitate (DNR) order completion (AOR, 2.78; $p = 0.003$) and predicted lower rates of intensive, life-prolonging care near death (AOR, 0.20; $p = 0.036$).

Implications for nursing communication from this study include the following points: Patients are individuals and attentive listening is essential. Be sure to individualize spiritual care; do not make assumptions about the relationship of religion/spirituality of the patient to the patient's desire for intensive, life-prolonging measures.

References

Bowlby (1980). *Attachment and loss: Loss, sadness and depression* (Vol. 3). New York: Basic Books.

Campbell, M. L. (2008). *Nurse to nurse palliative care.* New York: McGraw-Hill.

Carson, V. B., & Koenig. H. G. (2004). *Spiritual caregiving: Healthcare as ministry.* West Conshohocken, PA: Templeton Press.

Ferrell, B. R., LaPorte Matzo, M., Penn, B., Sheehan, D. C., & Sherman, D. W. (2003). Communication skills for end-of-life nursing care: teaching strategies from the ELNEC curriculum *Nursing Education Perspectives, 24,* 4.

Jacobsen, J., Jackson, V., Dahlin, C., Greer, J., Perez-Cruz, P., Billings, J., ... Temel, J. (2011). Components of early outpatient palliative care consultation in patients with metastatic nonsmall cell lung cancer. *Journal of Palliative Medicine, 14*(4), 459–464. doi:10.1089/jpm.2010.0382

Koenig, H. G. (2008). *Medicine, religion and health.* West Conshohocken, PA: Templeton Press.

Kübler-Ross, E. (1969). *On death and dying.* London: Tavistock.

McSherry, W., & Ross, L. (2011). *Spiritual assessment in healthcare practice.* London: M & K Update.

Quality and Safety Education for Nurses. (2007). Pre-licensure knowledge, skills and attitudes. Retrieved from http://qsen.org/competencies/pre-licensure-ksas/#patient-centered_care

Rex Smith, A. (2006). Using the synergy model to provide spiritual care in critical care settings. *Critical Care Nurse, 26*(4), 41–47.

Rex Smith, A. (2007). Something more: Presence in nursing practice *Journal of Christian Nursing, 24*(2), 82–87.

Worden, J. W. (1991). *Grief counseling and grief therapy: A handbook for the mental health practitioner* (2nd ed.). New York: Springer.

CHAPTER SIXTEEN

Anger, Anxiety, and Difficult Communication Styles

Lisa Kennedy Sheldon

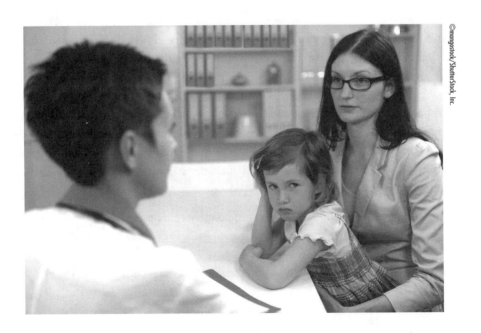

©mangostock/ShutterStock, Inc.

■ CASE STUDY

Mrs. R. arrives by wheelchair at the outpatient center for an intravenous infusion of zoledronic acid, a treatment for osteoporosis to prevent further deterioration of her bones. Unfortunately, the osteoporosis has been debilitating for Mrs. R. because of several fractures that have decreased her ability to walk and live independently. The nurse, who knows Mrs. R. from previous visits, arrives in the waiting room to bring Mrs. R. back for her infusion.

> *Nurse*: "Good morning, Mrs. R. Are you ready to get started?"
>
> *Mrs. R.*: "Ready? What good does this do me? You think I want to have this?"
>
> *Nurse*: "You sound upset today."
>
> *Mrs. R.*: "You don't know what it's like. I am just another patient to you. Get them in and get them out, right?"

Introduction

Not every patient is easy to deal with or grateful for nursing care. The stress brought on by changes in health and the demands of illness can disrupt a patient's normal ways of interacting with people. Additionally, previous life experiences, family and social relationships, and personality factors can all affect how patients respond to changes in health. Sometimes, patients say things that can be difficult to tolerate or even are offensive to nurses. This chapter discusses some situations that may make communication more challenging and presents some strategies for dealing with common patient responses to health, illness, and crisis. There are seven goals of nursing communication during difficult interactions:

1. Remain calm while acknowledging patient responses.
2. Demonstrate respect for the patient.
3. Promote patient control and autonomy.
4. Assess patient responses within the context of the current situation and patient history.
5. Perform the necessary nursing interventions.

6. Evaluate patient responses and adjust communication.
7. Offer support and, if necessary, referral for further care.

Difficult Interactions

Patients respond in a variety of ways to changes in health, especially during unexpected illness, trauma, or diminished functioning. You may find it easy to talk with some patients, whereas others may not be as open, which can make interactions more difficult. Other patients may readily express strong negative emotions such as anger and hostility. Some emotions expressed by patients are perceived as more difficult by nurses, provoking emotional reactions *in nurses* (Sheldon, Barrett, & Ellington, 2006). Some common difficult interactions include patient expressions of strong emotions such as anger, anxiety, and depression, as well as responses to crisis. An understanding of these situations and some strategies can help nurses select effective responses based on the patient's needs.

Anger

Expressions of patient anger do not arise routinely during nursing care and they may come as a surprise. Anger is a human response to many situations, including frustration, as seen in this chapter's case study. Regardless of their origins, expressions of anger can be uncomfortable, especially for the person on the receiving end of the outburst. Until the source of the anger is identified, it may be difficult, even anxiety producing, for nurses to deal with patients who appear angry or hostile.

A patient could be angry for any number of reasons. Anger might be the patient's response to loss of control or loss of independence, both of which are common problems in hospital settings. These psychiatric issues may prompt feelings of anger that require more advanced care (see a textbook on psychiatric and mental health nursing). Anger may be a defensive reaction to asking the patient too much personal information. Anger might also be part of how a particular personality deals with stress or it may indicate depression. It could even be a response to similar, unresolved situations from the past. A patient might be fearful of the illness and treatment or uncertain about the future. There are many causes of anger, requiring the nurse to pause and assess each situation as a unique scenario.

Unfortunately, anger may also be misdirected, especially during stressful situations. It may be displaced onto the nurse—that is, anger may be directed at the nurse but actually arise from other causes. Alternatively, the patient might actually be angry about circumstances arising out of the healthcare experience. For example, a patient in severe pain who has been waiting more than an hour for pain medication might yell at the nurse. Because of the variety of sources, anger must be understood as a human response to a stressful situation and assessed individually to understand the patient's behavior and identify the source of the concerns.

Anger is a complex emotion. Trying to understand what generated an angry response requires active listening during the outburst, which is not always a simple job. For the nurse to remain calm while acknowledging responses that arise internally requires self-knowledge, experience, and maturity. When the nurse remains calm, the emotional component of the patient's message is verbalized and then allowed to dissipate prior to the nurse's response. At the same time, listening calmly for the actual content of the message may reveal the origins of the anger. Patients need to be heard when they are angry, and the best approach is often to listen first and focus on their needs. Then, reflection and restatement or clarification may be used to validate and expand what was heard. It is important for the nurse to listen without becoming defensive or withdrawing, both of which are common responses to anger. Also, it is natural to want to avoid dealing with further anger or feeling personally attacked. Most of the time, the patient needs to express anger as part of the process of coping with the situation. Occasionally, the nurse's behavior or lack of action may be the source of the anger. If the nurse's responses or actions (or lack of action, as in the example of the delayed pain medication) have prompted the patient's anger, then active listening is still the best approach followed by an apology, if appropriate.

There are several ways to work through angry interactions with patients (Box 16-1). First, the nurse should suspend personal responses to angry outbursts. It may be difficult not to react to a patient's anger, but it is an important first step in addressing the situation. This requires taking a deep breath, relaxing, and calmly listening to the content of the patient's message. Common responses from nurses to patients' anger include disliking the patient or feeling angry or defensive when dealing with the patient. These responses might result from the nurse's personal life experiences with anger. However, the nurse should allow the patient to express his or her concerns and the emotion associated with the message.

Patients often experience changes in normal communication patterns when confronted with illness.

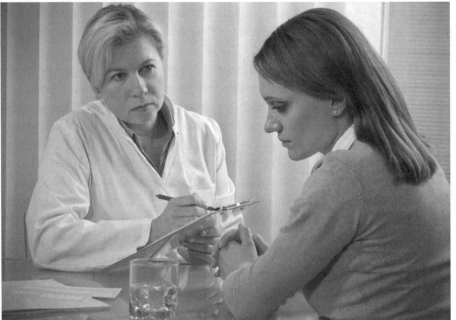

© iStockphoto/Thinkstock

Box 16-1 Dealing with Expressions of Anger

- Listen, stay calm, and let the patient set the pace.
- Avoid becoming defensive, withdrawn, or aggressive during the outburst.
- Keep the tone of voice low and controlled, speaking softly and slowly.
- Avoid excessive smiling or rote responses.
- Reflect or restate what has been said, seeking clarification.
- Acknowledge the emotional component of the message.
- Pause after the outburst to allow the emotional energy to dissipate.
- Offer to work with the patient to solve the problem.
- Use clear, assertive ("I") responses about possible actions to resolve the problem.
- Seek assistance promptly if the situation is escalating, the patient is unable to control his or her anger, and/or there is a threat of physical harm.

Sometimes a pause and silence are necessary to allow the emotion to dissipate and permit both the nurse and the patient to gather their thoughts prior to responding.

Once the patient's concerns are expressed, the nurse can begin to resolve the situation. The first step is to ask the patient for clarification of their concerns using restatement or reflection. For example, suppose a patient rings the call bell and yells at the nurse manager, saying he has been waiting for at least an hour for his pain medicine. The nurse could respond, "You have been waiting too long for your pain medicine. Is that right?"

The second step is acknowledgment of the emotional component of the patient's message. For example, the nurse could respond to the patient by saying, "You are already uncomfortable and this situation is frustrating." This provides confirmation that the nurse understands what the patient is experiencing and may serve to decrease the patient's anger.

Finally, the nurse can devise appropriate solutions to resolve the issues. The use of "We" statements lets the patient know that the nurse understands the situation and will work with the patient to resolve the situation. For example, the nurse could say, "I want to make sure that, in the future, you receive your pain medicine within 15 minutes of your request. We can. . . ." When the nurse offers to work together with the patient to solve the problem, the patient regains some control over his or her environment and perceives support from the nurse in resolving the problems.

For patients who have psychiatric diagnoses or who are under the influence of drugs, expressions of anger may require more intensive management and treatment. In such cases, anger may escalate into aggression, hostility, and physical violence against the nurse. Aggression is often defined as any verbal or nonverbal behavior that is threatening to or harms another. The most common settings for physical violence against nurses are emergency departments, psychiatric hospitals, and nursing homes. If a nurse senses that the patient is becoming more aggressive, cannot control his or her anger, or has the potential for violence, additional help should be sought at once. Safety of the nursing staff is an occupational obligation of the workplace, and additional assistance should always be available to protect the nursing staff and other patients. Nurses should also be familiar with and use the institution-specific policies and procedures (e.g., security response teams) to promote safety for everyone.

Anxiety

When patients are faced with threats to their health and well-being, a natural reaction is to become anxious. The feeling of anxiety might result from fear, frustration, conflict, or as a common response to stress and the unknown. Anxiety is an uncomfortable feeling of dread or apprehension, and the source of the feeling may or may not be known. Anxiety can occur with different levels of intensity. Low-level anxiety may actually increase mental and physical functioning and memory. Conversely, as the level of anxiety increases, awareness and interaction with the environment decreases, impairing recall and functioning.

- **Mild anxiety** is common in daily life and can be productive, even helpful, in meeting life's challenges. For example, mild anxiety can actually improve performance on an exam.
- **Moderate anxiety** may cause a decreased level of awareness and a diminished ability to pay attention. For example, the patient might not remember preoperative teaching before major surgery if he or she is experiencing moderate anxiety. It may be helpful to have another person, such as a family member, accompany the patient to the preoperative visit. Also, providing written instructions will help to reinforce the teaching and serve as a reminder for the patient after the visit.
- **Severe anxiety** produces a significantly decreased ability to focus and interact with the environment except for a few details. Increased anxiety levels can produce physical symptoms such as heart palpitations, sweating, dry mouth, bowel disturbances, and sleep disturbances. If the anxiety further intensifies, panic may develop, accompanied by severe incapacitation and inability to function.

Nurses are often called upon to identify and reduce anxiety in their patients (Box 16-2). Signs and symptoms of anxiety may include restlessness, tremors, hand wringing, forgetfulness, difficulty sleeping, rapid breathing, and heart palpitations. Excessive use of the call bell and repetitive questions are examples of patient behaviors that could signify higher levels of anxiety. Identification of the source of anxiety can lead to appropriate interventions.

SIGNS AND SYMPTOMS OF ANXIETY

Psychological Symptoms

Recurrent thoughts about diagnosis and treatment

Concerns about changes in functioning and roles

Fears about the future

Worries about death

Hypervigilance and scanning

Difficulty concentrating

Box 16-2 Strategies for Helping Anxious Patients

- Be alert to signs and symptoms of anxiety.

- Try to understand the patient's feelings by demonstrating a sincere desire to help the patient.

- Avoid becoming tense or defensive if the patient starts complaining or expressing anger.

- Speak slowly and briefly, avoiding rote phrases such as "Just pull yourself together" or "You'll feel better tomorrow."

- Help the patient verbalize his or her feelings and try to identify the source of anxiety.

- Do not assume the cause of the patient's anxiety without validating it with the patient. Sometimes patients cannot identify the cause but anxiety still exists.

- Assess the patient's support systems.

- Identify previously useful coping mechanisms.

- Offer explanations or information appropriate to the patient and the situation.

- Tailor interventions to alleviate the source of anxiety where possible or support the patient through the situation.

- Refer patients with severe and/or unresolved anxiety for further evaluation.

Physical Symptoms

Tachycardia or palpitations

Sweating

Perception of dyspnea or shortness of breath

Headaches

Restlessness and fidgeting

Abdominal distress

Loss of appetite

Nurses are not immune to anxiety, and many situations in health care are very stressful. Anxiety is a very contagious emotion. It is helpful if nurses understand, on a personal level, what triggers their own anxiety. For example, some nurses find performing painful procedures on patients, such as changing burn dressings, very stressful. If this is the case, it might help to talk with peers, role-play or review procedures to build confidence, and alternate patient assignments to decrease work-related anxiety and decrease the impact on patient care. Also, nurses intervene more therapeutically with patients when they can separate their personal responses from the patients' reactions. This requires self-knowledge and a variety of clinical experiences. This process may also preserve nurses' psychological well-being, decrease emotional burnout, and increase job satisfaction.

Some of the best approaches to reducing patient anxiety are already part of the nursing role. For example, nurses have flexible communication styles that they adapt to different patients and situations. They have a variety of communication skills: assessing patients' personalities and response to situations, interpreting different health problems, teaching self-care strategies, answering questions, explaining medications and side effects, and frequently negotiating the healthcare system to advocate for their patients' needs. Often, nurses use different educational techniques to diffuse anxiety about the unknown and decrease patient distress. Nurses provide supportive and compassionate care during stressful events such as surgery (see the evidence-based article on the effects of music on anxiety during operative procedures at the end of the chapter) or facilitate the decision-making process. In addition, nurses can often identify what patients perceive as threatening, assess the patients' support systems and previous coping mechanisms, and plan interventions to alleviate anxiety. Sometimes what patients need is to talk and share their perspectives, and active listening by a nurse may be a therapeutic way to diminish patients' anxiety.

Depression

The patient who appears to be depressed is always a concern to the nurse. Some depressive symptoms are short-term, normal responses to changes in health, relationships, or circumstances. For example, the patient with diabetes who has a limb amputated because of circulatory impairment will naturally be saddened by the loss of mobility and change in body image and lifestyle. Nurses' approach to the depressive symptoms in this patient will be different from interventions with a patient with a long-standing diagnosis of depression (Box 16-3).

Feelings of sadness are not the same thing as depression. Many patients and families experience sadness during loss of function, diminished health and well-being, or as part of the grieving process. For example, the loss of a loved one, major changes in life situation, or the diagnosis of a life-shortening illness may all cause feelings of sadness, hopelessness, futility, and helplessness. Signs and symptoms of depression, however, may include changes in appetite and sleep habits, lack of interest in previous activities, decreased libido, crying, and slowed speech and movement. Depressive symptoms may occur as part of the normal grieving process or due to *situational depression*. However, prolonged sadness (lasting for more than 2 weeks) with changes in normal functioning may indicate significant depression and require further assessment, referral, and treatment. In contrast, situational depression is time limited, the patient's symptoms will gradually lift, and the patient will begin to resume his or her normal life activities.

More severe depression lasts longer than situational depression and may or may not have a basis in a disturbing life event. Patients with severe depression often have low energy levels and little interest in daily activities. They may have feelings of worthlessness, hopelessness, and futility. One great concern for healthcare providers is that these feelings may lead to suicidal ideation as a way to put an end to the suffering. Depressed patients who become increasingly withdrawn, agitated, or restless, or who talk about killing themselves, even jokingly, require immediate intervention. While most patients who express sadness are not suicidal, nurses should be aware of the warning signs and not hesitate to refer patients for more intensive evaluation and treatment.

Refer to a text on psychiatric and mental health nursing for the best strategies for working with patients with a history of depression or suicidal tendencies. In addition, nurses should make appropriate referrals within their agencies or to other mental healthcare professionals.

Simple assessment of depression can be a part of nursing evaluation (Box 16-3). Fortin , Dwamena, Framkel, and Smith (2012) recommend two questions:

Over the last 2 weeks are you:

1. Having little interest or pleasure in doing things?
2. Feeling down, depressed, or hopeless?

If the patient answers "yes" to either question and identifies the frequency as "nearly every day" or "more than half the days," then the nurse should refer the patient for further assessment and/or treatment (pp. 100–101).

Box 16-3	Talking with Depressed Patients

- Initiate the conversation ("You seem unhappy").

- Show understanding, caring, and acceptance of behaviors, including tears and anger.

- Focus on the patient's abilities, promoting a realistic and hopeful attitude.

- Discourage the patient from making any major life decisions.

- Encourage simple activities (such as gardening, folding laundry) as the depression starts to lift.

- Take seriously all suicidal ideas and statements (like "ending it" or "doing myself in" or "showing them"); begin immediate interventions to promote patient safety and refer the patient to the appropriate professional for evaluation and treatment.

Crisis Situations

A crisis can occur whenever the normal balance of life is disturbed and usual coping skills are inadequate. Arnold and Boggs (2011) define two broad categories of crises: developmental and situational (pp. 460–461).

Developmental crises occur during normal growth and development. From birth to death, normal milestones present challenges to functioning and opportunities for growth. Examples of developmental crises include weaning, starting school or college, marriage, divorce, birth of a child, retirement, and death of a loved one. Erikson (1963) described developmental milestones as a series of crises that upset the normal balance, requiring new strategies to mature through the crisis. Successful negotiation of a developmental crisis allows restoration of equilibrium and continued growth.

Whereas developmental crises are frequently interwoven into other life events, *situational crises* arise out of external events over which a person has no control. When a situation is unexpected, it can produce stress as the patient tries to adapt using his or her available resources and previously successful coping strategies. A crisis develops when the patient's usual coping abilities are overwhelmed by the unplanned event. Examples of situational crises include sudden illness, work-related injury, house fire, or a car accident.

Both types of crises result in predictable phases of behavior. Fink (1986) described the phases as shock, defensive retreat, acknowledgment (renewal stress), adaptation, and change. The shock phase begins when the patient is first faced with the event. The patient might feel that the event is unreal and soon after feel bewildered. Suggestions from others are most helpful at this time before the patient moves into the next phase.

In the second phase, defensive retreat, the patient tries to reduce the sense of overwhelming stress with denial, anger, or wishful thinking. During the third phase, acknowledgment, the patient admits the reality of the situation and begins to mobilize resources and coping skills to adapt to the situation. If this phase is not successfully navigated, apathy and negative outcomes, such as depression, may develop.

In the final phase, adaptation and change, the patient regains a sense of self in a changed reality. Anxiety and tension often decrease during this phase, and patients welcome help from outside sources as they move forward in their life.

Nursing interventions during crises focus on the patient's situation and past experiences, previously effective coping skills, and current circumstances (Box 16-4). The nursing assessment should include the following elements:

- The event and its effect on the patient and family
- Available support systems
- Previous coping skills used by the patient during stressful situations
- Risk assessment for suicidal or violent behavior

Situational crises, such as injury, may strain the patient's usual coping abilities.

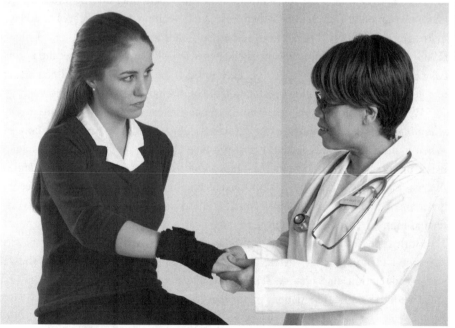

© Hemera/Thinkstock

Box 16-4	Interventions for Crisis Situations

- Establish a therapeutic relationship that facilitates open and effective communication.
- Allow the patient to express his or her feelings and talk about the events. This will help diminish tension.
- Assess coping behaviors that have worked for this patient. Review previous coping strategies and explore new ways of dealing with stressful events.
- Encourage the patient to seek and accept help from others, including significant others, religious affiliations, and community groups.
- Support the patient in the development of personal relationships to diminish stress and refocus the patient on the rewarding aspects of life.
- Refer patients for further evaluation and treatment if the crisis is overwhelming for the patient and/or if there is a risk for suicidal or violent behavior.

After the assessment, the goals of treatment are set with the patient and family. Nursing interventions are tailored to the individual patient and may include referral for further assessment and treatment. Interventions are aimed at reducing the impact of the stressful event and helping those affected by the event to learn new ways to cope with this crisis and future. James and Gilliland (2004) recommend a six-step model of crisis intervention:

1. *Ensure client safety.* Before intervening, make sure the client and others in the environment are safe.
2. *Define the problem.* Remain calm. Assess by active and reflective listening. Ask directed questions and use brief and simple responses. Identify emotional themes and prioritize problems.
3. *Provide support.* Provide compassionate support, but limit the number of providers. Normalize feelings, clarify concerns and distortions, and be truthful. Recognize clients' strengths. Use simple words and repeat them.
4. *Develop alternatives.* Develop options that give the client as much control as possible. Examine consequences, enlarge the perspective, and strengthen the client's natural support system.
5. *Make plans.* Help the client assume responsibility. Provide practical, short-term solutions, beginning with the present. Use previously effective

coping strategies; develop small, realistic goals; and stabilize community resources.

6. *Get commitment.* Set timelines, monitor achievement, and establish follow-up mechanisms.

Interviewing Difficulties

Often, during the interview and assessment process, nurses may find it difficult to obtain information from patients. Adequate data collection is an essential component of planning effective nursing care. Three common problems are vagueness, rambling discourse, and apathy.

Vagueness

Patients who are vague and do not share details about their health are often challenging to assess. Incomplete information also makes it difficult to accurately identify problems and nearly impossible to determine the necessary interventions. The causes of vagueness are varied and depend on the individual patient and the circumstances. Sometimes patients are vague because of a lack of understanding or mental acuity or due to the effects of medication or health conditions. Other patients may give vague answers when they are asked questions that they view as too intrusive, overly broad, anxiety-producing, or difficult to understand. When patients respond with vague answers, directed, closed-ended questions are often needed to elicit more specific information.

Patients may also give vague responses when they have difficulty understanding the medical terms used by healthcare providers or have low health literacy. At the beginning of the interaction, nurses can give patients permission to interrupt their conversation to ask the meaning of terms they do not understand. Also, if nurses use colloquial words and phrases instead of medical terms, patients may better understand the content of the conversation. For example, a patient might not understand the word "anticoagulant" but might understand the more commonly used phrase "blood thinner." Again, the flexibility of nursing communication skills will be valuable in tailoring the conversation to the individual patient.

If patients are anxious, they may not be able to focus on the interview or generate specific answers. If patients are vague in their responses to nurses' questions, then it may be necessary to reassess their concerns and anxiety levels prior to proceeding with the assessment. Nurses can pause and reestablish rapport, convey a sincere desire to help the patient, and try to identify and alleviate sources of anxiety (Box 16-5).

Box 16-5 Hints for Focusing Vague Answers

- Ensure that a trusting relationship has been established.
- Assess the patient's understanding, including level of consciousness, hearing, mental acuity, and anxiety level.
- Use general, open-ended questions such as "How can I help you today?" or "Which concerns do you have today?"
- Use directed and detailed questions to help the patient focus. "Tell me more about the . . . (specific symptom or concern)."
- Assure the patient the right to privacy. Preface sensitive questions with "Some people feel uncomfortable talking about . . ."
- Remember that the interview may be vague or difficult, not the patient.

Vagueness may also result when patients feel threatened or do not want to divulge personal or sensitive information. If a patient feels threatened or uncomfortable, the nurse may want to reassess whether trust has been established and restate the goals of the interaction. Even then, there may be subjects the patient does not want to discuss, feels ashamed of, or even worries how the nurse will react. Nurses can reaffirm their nonjudgmental concern and respect for patients, relieving potential shame or guilt associated with self-revelation. They may also need to reiterate that shared information is confidential, within legal boundaries, and used to improve their care. If the nurse's questions seem to be increasing the patient's anxiety or the details are not necessary for the patient's immediate care, the nurse may want to stop, acknowledge the patient's right to privacy, and proceed to other aspects of the assessment.

Rambling

Rambling conversation may be informative but frequently may become less focused on the current patient needs. While these conversations may be entertaining, they can hinder timely assessments and nursing care delivery. Sometimes, rambling interactions can prolong data collection and result in unfocused and inefficient care. While some personalities are apt to be more talkative, it is important to remember that excessive talking may also indicate high anxiety levels or cognitive impairment. Keeping the interview focused on the goals of the interaction and the patient's health concerns will provide more accurate data in a timely manner (Box 16-6). Nurses should use information in the patients' interview to

Box 16-6	Dealing with Rambling

- Help the patient focus on the topic at hand: "I'd enjoy talking about this, but let's return to . . ." or "I'd like to hear more about . . ."
- Clarify what you heard with the patient: "I think you said that . . ."
- Reestablish the purpose of the visit: "Today we need to focus on . . ."

redirect back to the purpose of the interactions. Later, as time permits, interesting conversations about the patient's experiences may provide more detailed information and often enrich the nurse–patient relationship.

Apathy

Working with patients who are apathetic or unmotivated is challenging for nurses. Many patients come to healthcare providers to change their behaviors or to help them adopt healthier lifestyles, while others need to make changes to become healthier. One counseling style, known as motivational interviewing (MI), was developed by Miller and Rollnick (2002) to address reluctance to change. Using a nonjudgmental, nonconfrontational, and nonadversial approach, MI uses four steps to help patients consider making change:

1. Express empathy so counselors (nurses) understand the patient's experience.
2. Develop the discrepancy between where the patient is now and where they want to be or between their values and the reality.
3. Roll with resistance because reluctance to change is a normal—not pathological—response.
4. Support self-efficacy and patient autonomy to move forward confidently.

MI is described as a client-centered, goal-directed approach to help patients make change. It has been used in the treatment of alcohol abuse and smoking cessation as well as to address mental health issues and adherence to treatment regimens. Training programs are available (see the list of websites at the end of the chapter).

Difficult Behaviors

Not all interactions with patients are simple or manageable. Sometimes, patients express an array of behaviors that some nurses may find challenging to handle. Difficult interactions often create emotional responses in nurses, which can impede their ability to make clear judgments and create therapeutic responses. Having an understanding of some common difficult scenarios prepares nurses for handling these situations so that they are less surprising and more manageable. Two common types of difficult behaviors are patients who are demanding and those displaying sexually overt behaviors.

Demanding Behavior

When independent people are put in the position of dependency and uncertainty, they often feel threatened and may become demanding of the staff. As patients, these people may relate to nurses with simple responses and repeated requests for services, perhaps because of increased anxiety levels or out of a need for more control over the environment. They may feel less threatened if they can maintain some control over unpredictable situations or participate in decision making about their treatment or schedule. Sometimes their repeated demands may make nurses feel inadequate or even subservient. In turn, responses by nurses to demanding patients are often defensive ones. Unfortunately, such defensive behaviors by nurses are likely to result in stilted conversations with little meaningful content. Nurses may respond or be tempted to avoid demanding patients, which can further patients' views of receiving less care or attention and even less control. This vicious cycle can lead to poor nurse–patient relationships, hurried assessments, and inadequate nursing care that can affects patient outcomes.

The best responses by nurses to demanding behaviors will incorporate a calm, neutral approach and supportive care (Box 16-7). To remain emotionally neutral, nurses may need to pause and collect themselves before responding to patients. By not taking offense or relating emotionally to demanding remarks, the nurse can understand the patient's perspective. The nurse may try using a flexible communication style and acknowledging the patient's concerns by restating and summarizing. When the patient has expressed his or her concerns or needs, the nurse may then provide the patient with explanations about available resources and time. At that point, the nurse can offer to work with the patient to meet his or her needs using the available resources. Nursing interventions that are geared toward mutually established goals help the patient regain control and assist the nurse in delivering efficient care to all the patients. Limit setting that is consistently applied by all the involved staff may be necessary if the patient's requests are extensive or burdensome to the staff. Once a plan is in place to meet the patient's needs, it is essential that the nurse and team follow up with the plan. This helps to build trust with the patient and shows respect for the individual.

Box 16-7	Some Approaches to Demanding Patients

- Take a deep breath and listen.
- Avoid a defensive response.
- Talk in a moderate tone of voice.
- Do not engage in debating, but rather be inquisitive and flexible.
- Explain the nurse's role and availability to the patient.
- Incorporate the patient's wishes as permitted by time and resources.
- Seek support from peers so that patient care is not compromised.
- Set limits as necessary to ensure safe and effective care for all patients.

Sexually Overt Behavior

All human beings are sexual beings. To deny the existence of sexuality is to limit the human experience. In Maslow's hierarchy of needs, sexuality is one of the basic needs, similar to food, air, and water. When patients enter the healthcare setting, they do not become asexual. That is, while they might wear unisex gowns and identification bands, they do not have their sexuality locked away with their valuable possessions. The experience of illness and disability can change how patients express and maintain their sexuality. Nursing assessments and interventions that address issues of sexuality need to be thoughtful and careful, acknowledging the patient's right to privacy while providing the necessary care (Box 16-8).

Physical touch is an important part of nursing care such as bathing or assisting with ambulation or repositioning, However, it can be misunderstood by some patients, or patients may feel very uncomfortable with needing and receiving such personal care. Patients may make sexually explicit remarks, demonstrate inappropriate touching, or make jokes that are uncomfortable for nurses, such that nurses may be reluctant to spend time with them. Nurses should respond respectfully, honestly, and immediately to address inappropriate comments or touching to set limits and explain the professional intent and necessity of the physical care (Box 16-9). If this direct approach is ineffective, then nurses should discuss the matter with supervisors, social workers, and/or psychiatry departments to develop strategies for limiting patient behavior while providing the necessary care.

| **Box 16-8** | Basic Rules for Communicating About Sexuality |

- Maintain privacy in the physical space (closed doors and curtains).
- Reveal private patient information only as needed to those involved in the patient's care (see HIPAA guidelines).
- Avoid making judgments about the patient's decisions, lifestyle, or values.
- Prevent shameful or embarrassing situations by providing for privacy, assessing patient readiness to talk, and referring the patient to other healthcare providers for discussions regarding sexual issues that may not be comfortable for some nurses.
- Watch for cues that might indicate emotional scars from abuse, such as feelings of shame, aversion, or aggression.
- Do not assume that most adults know about sexual functioning and reproductive health.

| **Box 16-9** | Responding to Sexually Overt Behavior |

- Dress appropriately for the work environment.
- Monitor behavior and conversation to maintain professional boundaries.
- Respond immediately to inappropriate sexual talk or touch: "I prefer that you not touch me in that way" or "That kind of joke makes me uncomfortable."
- Set appropriate limits if patient behavior is repetitive: "If you talk that way again, your privileges will be taken away."
- Ask another nurse to be present during physical care or change patient assignments as needed to provide relief.
- Review the circumstances with trusted colleagues or supervisors.
- Collaborate with other healthcare providers for additional approaches and support.

Nurses need to be aware that their behaviors may also be misinterpreted by patients. Inappropriately fitting or revealing clothing or talking about personal details of one's life might confuse patients and blur the lines of the professional relationship between nurses and patients (see the section on self-disclosure in the *Interviewing Skills: A Clinical Art and Science* chapter). It is important to remember that the focus of the nurse–patient relationship is always *the patient*. When a nurse is unsure if a conversation or behavior is appropriate, the advice of a trusted colleague or supervisor may provide necessary feedback and suggest different approaches to working with the patient.

Summary

Patients are often stressed by changes in their health and functioning. The strain of a crisis can disrupt a patient's normal way of interacting with people, making nursing communication more difficult. Nurses may react personally to strong patient emotions such as anger and sadness. Understanding potentially challenging interactions prepares nurses to anticipate and decide on effective responses to patients and to be aware of their own responses. Specific strategies are helpful in working with patients during difficult interactions. The goal of these interactions is to maintain the personal integrity of both the patient and the nurse, understand and address the patient's needs or concerns, facilitate patient coping with changes in health, and provide therapeutic, effective, and timely nursing care.

Case Study Resolution

The nurse continued to wheel Mrs. R. back to a more private location and said, "Let's go back to a quieter spot to talk." Sitting in a chair beside Mrs. R., the nurse said, "Mrs. R., you are not just another patient to me. You seem upset today." With a sideways glance at the nurse, Mrs. R. responded, "I was once young like you. I could walk and take care of myself. Now, I wake up and I check on what hurts today. I have to be so careful. Life just isn't fun anymore." The nurse paused, put her hand on Mrs. R.'s hand and asked, "What can I do to help?"

EXERCISES

Working in groups of three, pick one of the following three scenarios to act out. One person will be the "patient," one the "nurse," and one the "observer." Taking 10 minutes, act out the scenario.

1. Mrs. P. is a 68-year-old woman admitted to the medical–surgical floor for a thoracotomy tomorrow. Four weeks ago she was on the same floor for a lung biopsy, which proved positive for a non-small-cell lung cancer. Today she has made nasty remarks to the admitting nurse about the quality of care at the hospital and she has been standing in her doorway, across from the nursing station, for the last hour, staring at the nurses.

2. Mr. G. is a 44-year-old man with multiple myeloma who is in the outpatient unit for a monthly infusion. The nurse, a 28-year-old woman, enters the

room, and the patient says, "My, aren't we looking sexy today. You look better every time I come here." When she starts to take his blood pressure, he pats her knee.

3. Sr. R. is a 72-year-old nun and elementary school teacher. She comes into the ambulatory care clinic with a cough. The triage nurse is interviewing the patient to get more details about her past medical history and current symptoms. Sr. R. very sweetly starts to answer the questions but quickly starts telling stories about children she has taught in the past.

After the group enacts the chosen scenario, the observer will comment on the "nurse's" approaches to the "patient." Answer the following questions as a group:

- Which approaches diffused the situation?
- Which comments were not helpful to the patient?
- Which alternative approaches could be used in this situation?
- How does the nurse not react personally to some of the more challenging patients?
- Which resources are available to help the nurse deal with these situations?

Websites

American Academy on Communication in Healthcare. Teaching Modules (15-day free trial and subscription): Working with Patients with Anxiety/Panic Disorders and Depression.

http://www.aachonline.org/doccom/
Motivational Interviewing Network of Trainers (MINT)
http://motivationalinterview.org/training/trainers.html

Evidence-Based Article

Mok, E., & Wong, K. Y. (2003). The effects of music on patient anxiety. *Association of Perioperative Registered Nurses, 77*(2), 396–410.

Surgery under local anesthesia can be anxiety producing for patients. In this study, patients selected music to listen to during surgery under local anesthesia. The researchers measured patients' vital signs and reported anxiety before and after surgery. They found that patients who listened to their choice of music during the procedure had significantly lower levels of anxiety, lower heart rate, and lower blood pressure as compared to patients who did not listen to music.

References

Arnold, E. C., & Boggs, K. U. (2011). Communicating with clients in crisis. (pp. 413–436.) In E. C. Arnold & K. U. Boggs (Eds.), *Interpersonal relationships: Professional communication skills for nurses* (6th ed.). St. Louis, MO: Elsevier Saunders.

Erikson, E. (1963). *Childhood and society.* New York: Norton.

Fink, S. (1986). *Crisis management: Planning for the inevitable.* Watertown, MA: American Medical Associates.

Fortin, A. H., Dwamena, F. C., Framkel, R. M., & Smith, R. C. (2012). 5-step patient-centered interviewing. In *Smith's patient-centered interviewing: An evidence-based method* (p. 30). New York: McGraw-Hill.

James, R., & Gilliland, B. (2004). *Crisis intervention strategies* (5th ed.). Belmont, CA: Thomson Books/Cole.

Miller, W. R., & Rollnick, S. (2002). *Motivational interviewing: Preparing people to change* (2nd ed.). New York: Guilford Press.

Sheldon, L. K., Barrett, R., & Ellington, L. (2006). Difficult communication in nursing. *Journal of Scholastic Nursing, 38*(2), 141–147.

CHAPTER SEVENTEEN

Compassion Fatigue: Caring for Yourself

Lisa Kennedy Sheldon

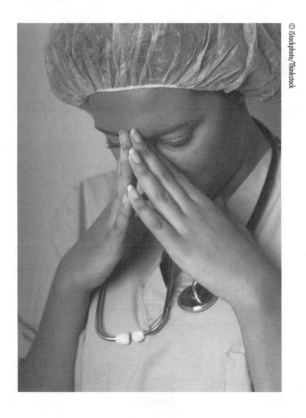

© iStockphoto/Thinkstock

■ CASE STUDY

Sally has been working on the medical–surgical unit for almost 14 years. She has seen everything—treatment successes and medication mistakes, healing patients and grieving families. Over the years, she has worked with great colleagues as well as nurses and doctors who have been difficult to work with. Sally used to get involved with patients, even going to their homes to do follow-up visits, but now they are discharged so quickly that she barely has time to get to know them. Right now, Sally feels that no matter how much she does to care for her patients, she has never done enough. In addition, she has other responsibilities at home with her family.

Today, Sally is caring for a young man who has developed a fever after chemotherapy for Hodgkin's lymphoma. He is very concerned about the potential of a serious infection. He asks Sally about the results of his blood counts this morning. She replies, "I don't know. Don't worry about that. Let's just get your vital signs—that's important."

Spectrum of Compassion

Nurses respond to patients' needs by providing healing, comfort, and support in addition to physical care. They elicit patient concerns so that they can understand their patients' needs. These compassionate behaviors demonstrate care and concern for others. Compassionate care by nurses is often described with four terms: altruism, sympathy, compassion, and empathy. Further definition of these terms provides different perspectives on approaches to responding to patients and providing personalized, patient-centered care.

- *Altruism* is defined as understanding of the experience of another involving self-sacrifice or putting the good of another before yourself.
- *Sympathy* is sharing or experiencing the feelings of another person.
- *Compassion* is the desire to understand the experience of another person accompanied by a desire to relieve suffering.
- *Empathy* includes a broader definition that may be more compatible with the goals of nursing: educated compassion or intellectual understanding of the emotional state of another. Empathy is the sincere showing of concern, a desire to understand, and the goal of relieving suffering while providing professional assessment and interventions.

There probably exists a spectrum of compassion. At its best, professional compassion contains elements of an empathetic desire to understand another's experience and a compassionate goal to alleviate suffering. When merged with professional standards, compassion and empathy direct nursing care through a desire to understand suffering and a call to act to foster patient comfort and well-being.

Compassion is empathy in action.

Compassion, Fatigue, and Burnout

If empathy involves a desire to understand the patient's experience and compassion combines empathy with the intent to help, then *compassion is empathy in action*. Action, of course, requires effort and work. When nurses continue to help and work with patients without caring for themselves, they become at risk for burnout. The work of nursing entails much more than just physical and technical care; it requires emotional work and often difficult communication (Sheldon, Barrett, & Ellington, 2006). Because nurses respond to a variety of patient concerns during the course of routine care, they are also witnesses to situations that may be extremely sad or desperate or violent. Emotional situations may arise spontaneously, even at surprising times. Watching and responding to patient suffering exacts a toll that requires processing by nurses. Eifried (2003) describes the experience of bearing witness to patient suffering and the toll it may take on nursing students. This experience is not unique to students, however, and often even experienced nurses are surprised by their emotional reactions to patient situations.

Burnout occurs quietly, building for months or years before nurses understand what is happening. Nurses may show changes in their lifestyles such as behaviors of excessive smoking, drinking, or eating; they may feel tired all the time or they may have difficulty falling or staying asleep. Emotionally, nurses experiencing burnout may become less emotionally accessible and have difficulty in their personal relationships. Conversely, they may actually become overly involved with their patients. They may work harder but feel more tired and less appreciated (Arnold & Boggs, 2007, pp. 452–453). Eventually, nurses with burnout may feel that the demands of their work exceed their resources and become dissatisfied with their work and look for another job. At its worst, burnout can also affect patient care and prevent the nurse from fully engaging with patients to minimize effort and involvement. Sometimes nurses distance themselves from patients in an effort to protect themselves. Consequences of such distance contribute to incomplete assessments, lack of responsiveness to patient concerns, and less effective nursing care.

Self-Care

How nurses care for themselves and their colleagues is vitally important to providing optimal, responsive, and effective nursing care. The stress of caring for others, witnessing painful situations, and handling difficult interactions all build cumulatively unless nurses take care of themselves. In the American Nurses Association Code of Ethics (2001), one tenet acknowledges that nurses need to care for themselves because of the unique nature of their job. The nurse owes the same duties to self as to others, including the responsibility to preserve integrity and safety, to maintain competence, and to continue personal and professional growth.

Strategies to promote rejuvenation vary by clinical setting and by individual nurse. For example, nurses in emergency departments may valiantly try to save the victims of a motor vehicle accident. If their efforts are not successful, they may need a debriefing to allow staff to air their feelings of frustration and loss and to provide support to one another. In contrast, the staff in an oncology unit may lose a long-term patient and organize a memorial service to honor the patient, express their grief, and provide closure.

Probably the most important form of support for nurses comes from their peers. Difficult situations arise spontaneously on patient care units, providing nurses with the ability to express their needs and for others to provide assistance on a more immediate basis. Collegial support and a team atmosphere may be the best protection against burnout and dissatisfaction with the job of nursing.

Self-care strategies may be individualized depending on the nurse but all require an awareness of the self. What is important is that nurses realize that their work may require additional sources of support and rejuvenation beyond other occupations. Exercise, relaxation breathing, meditation, yoga, massage, religious and spiritual connections, and positive relationships with family and friends are all examples of sources of rejuvenation that may help nurses cope with their jobs. Nursing management needs to build in strategies that acknowledge the emotional work of nursing and address the needs of nurses. By supporting themselves, nurses are enhancing the abilities of the nurses to be fully present with their patients, facilitate more thorough assessments, respond more effectively to patient concerns, and improve the quality of nursing care delivery.

Recovering from Burnout

Recovering from burnout requires careful reflection and self-awareness. Nurses should be honest in appraising their work environment and their responses to it. Trusted colleagues or friends may be able to provide direct observations and emotional support. Sometimes the goals are unrealistic or the nurse has too high expectations. In addition, nurses need to restore balance to their lives by making choices that improve job satisfaction. They need to be realistic about what they can accomplish in a day and set appropriate goals. By setting goals, they can separate work activities from their personal lives. With the separation of work and personal life, the nurse can take time to nurture the self with activities that are rejuvenating such as exercise, meditation, or outdoor activities.

Summary

Self-care strategies for nurses are necessary to enhance therapeutic relationships with patients. These strategies may also promote ongoing job satisfaction and create a better balance between the personal and professional dimensions of nursing care. Nurses can develop self-awareness and make positive life choices to improve their own health and well-being.

Case Study Resolution

Sally quickly took the vital signs and left the room to document them in the medical record. She paused and actually felt saddened by her response to her patient, realizing that she had been "cold" and technical in her care. She thought of her brother, who was close in age to this patient, and how she would like a nurse to talk with him if he were sick. Sally went back to the room and apologized for working too quickly this morning. She said, "I am sorry for being abrupt earlier. I know this has been a stressful time and you are worried about your blood counts. I will check the results and come back in 10 minutes. OK?"

Websites

5 Signs of Burnout. Monster.com

http://nursinglink.monster.com/benefits/articles/2481-5-signs-of-burnout

Evidence-Based Article

Kravits, K., McAllister-Black, R., Grant, M., & Kirk, C. (2010). Self care strategies for nurses: A psychoeducational intervention for stress reduction and the prevention of burnout. *Applied Nursing Research, 23*, 130–138.

The authors developed a 6-hour course to reduce stress and prevent burnout. In addition, the participants completed a wellness plan. The course included discussions about stress responses, coping patterns, the relaxation response, and guided imagery. It also included a section on art making. After attending the course, participants had lower scores on emotional exhaustion and higher scores on personal accomplishment. The authors recommend systematic efforts to promote nursing self-care behaviors and address work issues that increase burnout and emotional exhaustion.

References

Arnold, E. C., & Boggs, K. U. (2007). Effects of stress on the nurse. In *Interpersonal relationships: Professional communication skills for nurses* (5th ed., pp. 452–457). St. Louis, MO: Saunders Elsevier.

Eifried, S. (2003). Bearing witness to suffering: The lived experience of nursing students. *Nursing Education, 42*(2), 50–67.

Sheldon, L. K., Barrett, R., & Ellington, L. (2006). Difficult communication in nursing. *Journal of Nursing Scholarship, 38*(2), 141–147.

Communicating with Other Healthcare Providers

CHAPTER EIGHTEEN

Practicing Conflict Resolution, Negotiation, and Interprofessional and Intraprofessional Collaboration

JoAnn Mulready-Shick
Janice B. Foust

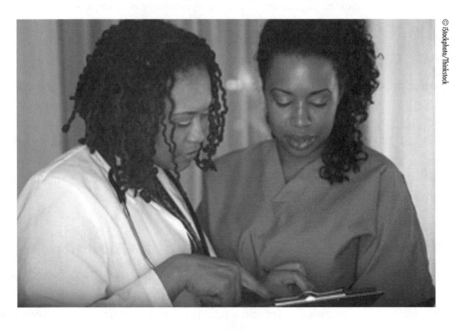

© iStockphoto/Thinkstock

■ CASE STUDY

It is the beginning of the evening shift and the newly licensed nurse, who recently completed orientation, is assigned to be the charge nurse on the rehabilitation unit. Given the staff mix on the unit for this shift, the charge nurse has also been assigned to administer intravenous (IV) medications. The charge nurse receives a report from a nursing staff member on Mrs. T., an 82-year-old widow who is receiving physical and occupational therapy for a left below-the-knee amputation and new prosthesis. Mrs. T. is now complaining of chest discomfort and a productive cough; a chest x-ray report, which was just communicated to the nurse, suggests pneumonia. The new charge nurse notices that no new orders were written during the day and decides to phone the resident on call with a patient update. The resident provides a telephone order to begin an IV antibiotic by saline lock.

One hour later, as the nurse starts the antibiotic, Mrs. T. is noticeably short of breath; the nurse provides the patient with oxygen and stops the medication. The nurse calls the resident to report that this patient's condition has worsened and needs closer monitoring. The nurse requests that the patient be evaluated for possible transfer to the subacute intensive care unit (ICU). The resident is irate that the nurse has called before completing the antibiotic administration and chastises the nurse further for making the transfer suggestion. The nurse is unsure how to respond.

Introduction

Nurses cite communication issues with physicians as an important contributing factor to patient care errors (Dingley, Daugherty, Derieg, & Persing, 2008). Intimidation has also been reported as a root cause of medication errors. In a study of 2000 healthcare professionals, half of the respondents reported feeling pressured into giving a medication for which they had questioned the safety but felt intimidated and unable to effectively communicate their concerns (Institute for Safe Medication Practices, 2004).

Nurse–Physician Communication Challenges

Nurse–physician communication can be challenging for a host of reasons, with many interrelated dynamics occurring simultaneously. Nurses are expected to communicate frequently with numerous medical providers.

Professionals from differing disciplines are involved with making decisions multiple times throughout the day and often from different locations, which collectively creates infrequent opportunities for routine interactions. Healthcare professionals inevitably hold their own disciplinary views about priority patient care needs and about the roles of members from other disciplines. Inherent in these differing perceptions of roles and responsibilities are issues of hierarchy, gender, educational preparation, culture, and formal and informal power. These differences concurrently produce conditions that are ripe for communication exchanges considered overbearing—namely, intimidation, inhibition, restraint, stereotyping, and fear—and can be harmful to patient care. Additional barriers to interprofessional communication and collaboration are listed in Box 18-1. How can nurses address such challenging conversations with medical staff and interact to promote greater trust, openness, and collaboration?

Healthcare team members work in environments where stress, fatigue, overload, time constraints, distractions, interruptions, and complex technologies are commonplace and often contribute to error formation. All too often, unrealistic expectations, blame, discontent, poor decision making, and patient harm can result from this potent mixture. In addition to errors in patient care, it is no wonder that nurse–physician communication is often named as an important cause of nurse job dissatisfaction (Larrabee et al., 2003).

In the chapter-opening case study, the new charge nurse's first response may have been surprise, annoyance, or disappointment. It appeared that the resident did not value the nurse's clinical judgment. Given the *Future of Nursing* report's recommendation for nurses to be full partners with physicians and other healthcare professionals and to practice to their highest potential (Institute of Medicine [IOM], 2011), it becomes clear that role clarification and collaboration among all team members has never been more important. In all healthcare settings, team members have a responsibility to create a milieu where all feel trust and respect for one another and are treated as equal and valued partners on the same team. Simultaneously, in the larger healthcare environment, teams of providers that include members from many disciplines and treat families and patients as equal partners are more likely to be rewarded with financial incentives for care coordination and chronic disease management. Teamwork, collaboration, and partnership imply understanding that diverse teams problem solve and make decisions better than

Box 18-1 Common Barriers to Interprofessional Communication and Collaboration

- Personal values and expectations
- Personality differences
- Hierarchy
- Disruptive behavior
- Culture and ethnicity
- Generational differences
- Gender
- Historical interprofessional and intraprofessional rivalries
- Differences in language and jargon
- Differences in schedules and professional routines
- Varying levels of preparation, qualifications, and status
- Differences in requirements, regulations, and norms of professional education
- Fears of diluted professional identity
- Differences in accountability, payment, and rewards
- Concerns regarding clinical responsibility
- Complexity of care
- Emphasis on rapid decision making

Source: Agency for Healthcare Research and Quality. (2013b). TeamSTEPPS® fundamentals course: Module 6—Communication. Retrieved from http://www.ahrq.gov/teamsteppstools/instructor/fundamentals/module6/igcommunication.htm

any one individual or group working alone. The time in which position and power dictated whose voices carried the most weight is now past—although not all healthcare team members are ready for, or have made, this transition. Healthcare improvement relies on the mutual goals of putting patient needs and teamwork first and valuing the contributions of all members. Unfortunately, the majority of healthcare professionals have not been educated in collaborative practices.

Leaders from various disciplines have come together to address this concern in a collective fashion. New graduates from health professional schools will be expected to practice from a set of common core competencies for improving quality and safety in today's complex healthcare systems. Not all practicing healthcare team members have acquired such skills nor have they learned, these shared competencies needed for collaborative, interprofessional practice. To address this issue, healthcare settings nowadays are providing learning opportunities for teams to be trained together in these core competencies, with the goal of continuing such interprofessional training throughout their careers. For improving teamwork and patient care quality, interprofessional education will start in school, but ongoing training will continue in workplaces. One model of such ongoing training is the Learning Continuum prelicensure through practice trajectory developed by the Interprofessional Education Collaborative (Figure 18-1).

Figure 18-1   Interprofessional Collaborative Practice Domains

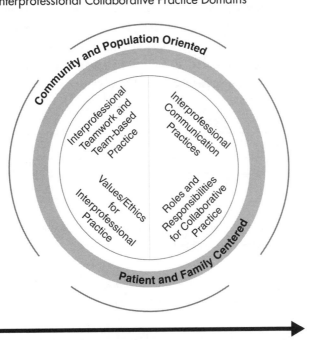

The Learning Continuum prelicensure through practice trajectory

Four domains of interprofessional collaborative practice were created in 2011 by the Interprofessional Education Collaborative (IPEC), a partnership of six associations—the American Association of Colleges of Nursing, the American Association of Colleges of Osteopathic Medicine, the American Association of Colleges of Pharmacy, the American Dental Education Association, the Association of American Medical Colleges, and the Association of Schools of Public Health. These involved professionals acknowledged their common concern for integrated, high-quality care for patients within the United States' current, evolving healthcare system. They identified a common set of competencies to advance substantive interprofessional learning experiences to prepare future clinicians for team-based care. The four domains identified for interprofessional collaborative practice are values and ethics, roles and responsibilities, communication, and teamwork (IPEC, 2011). (See Box 18-2).

In the chapter-opening case, shared values and understanding of roles and responsibilities, teamwork, and communication were not evident in the interaction between the charge nurse and the resident. Had these two professionals undergone interprofessional education or workplace training, this confrontation might not have occurred. Part of this shared learning for all team members involves learning strategies for negotiating disagreements and resolving conflict.

Box 18-2 | Interprofessional Collaborative Practice Domains

- *Assert values and ethics of interprofessional practice* by placing the interests, dignity, and respect of patients at the center of healthcare delivery and embracing the cultural diversity and differences of healthcare teams.

- *Leverage the unique roles and responsibilities of interprofessional partners* to appropriately assess and address the healthcare needs of patients and populations served.

- *Communicate with patients, families, communities, and other health professionals in support of a team approach* to preventing disease and disability, maintaining health, and treating disease.

- *Perform effectively in various team roles* to deliver patient/population-centered care that is safe, timely, efficient, effective, and equitable.

Adapted from Interprofessional Education Collaborative Expert Panel. (2011). *Core competencies for interprofessional collaborative practice: Report of an expert panel.* Washington, DC: Author.

Conflict Resolution Strategies

In the chapter-opening case study, the nurse's second response may have been an immediate urge to call the supervisor. However, when nurses become more accustomed to using assertive communication strategies conflicts can be more readily managed. Even so, conflict can be considered a normal occurrence and will intermittently occur whenever two persons are relating and expressing themselves. Nurses are faced with both interprofessional and intraprofessional conflicts on a regular basis that can impede teamwork and patient care. Therefore, conflict resolution and disagreement negotiation strategies are important collaborative communication competencies for all nurses to develop.

Often the same critical language that is helpful for speaking more assertively—particularly the Two-Challenge Rule and the CUS technique (both are discussed in the *Delegation and Assertive Communication* chapter)—can be useful when nurses encounter conflict. Another structured communication tool, known as the DESC script, can also be a helpful tool in conflict management and resolution (Agency for Healthcare Quality and Research [AHRQ], 2013a). The DESC script—**D**escribe, **E**xpress, **S**uggest **C**onsequences—is a useful strategy when other strategies are unsuccessful, when hostile or harassing behaviors recur, or when patient situations worsen (Box 18-3). Both hostile behavior and the possibility of a poor patient outcome were occurring in the chapter-opening case study.

In this case study, the nurse was confused, surprised, and likely unaccustomed to such confrontations. Nurses are also often "conflict averse" and may ignore opportunities to resolve conflicts or negotiate disagreements. In some situations, negotiation may be an important tactic for the nurse to use, particularly with

---

Box 18-3   DESC Script

Describe the specific situation or behavior and provide concrete evidence or data.

Express how the situation makes you feel and what your concerns are.

Suggest other alternatives and seek agreement.

Consequences should be stated in terms of impact on established team goals or patient safety.

Source: Agency for Healthcare Research and Quality. (2013a). TeamSTEPPS® fundamentals course: Module 5—Mutual support. Retrieved from http://www.ahrq.gov/teamsteppstools/instructor/fundamentals/module5/igmutualsupp.htm

nurse-to-nurse interactions. An effective negotiation response helps the nurse resolve situations when colleagues' needs and wants don't mesh. The aim of a win–win negotiation is to find a solution that is acceptable to both parties and that leaves both team members feeling that they've won or been respected and valued. In contrast, strategies such as forcing, competing, avoiding, compromising, accommodating and suppressing may be used in handling other conflict situations but may not result in a win–win outcome for both parties.

All nurses are expected to be skilled practitioners in interprofessional communication, which means that they must choose effective communication strategies and tools for facilitating discussions and interactions that enhance patient care and team functioning. In addition to daily use of these described communication strategies, nurses who participate in high-functioning teams are expected to give feedback to others about performance and respond respectfully as team members when receiving feedback from others. Learning to give and receive timely, sensitive, and instructive feedback with confidence helps health professionals improve their teamwork and team-based care. When nurses are members of a high-functioning team, constructive criticism is a valued component of team building. Patient safety and quality is always the team's priority. Additional group communication tools for high-functioning interprofessional team use include daily huddles, weekly patient safety meetings, multidisciplinary rounding, and rapid response teams.

Intraprofessional Communication

Nurse–nurse communication is also an essential step to promoting continuity of care and patient safety. Shift or transfer reports during hand-offs, when nurses transition responsibility for care, are frequently encountered examples of intraprofessional communication. Proactive nurse–nurse communication promotes patient safety. That is, nurses who share their clinical judgments, top priorities, and concerns help nurses receiving their reports to focus their care and alert them to potential complications. Another topic that helps nurses be more efficient is when they share strategies that are effective in working with individual patients (e.g., food preferences) as well as those that have not worked. Sharing this information helps nurses be more efficient (e.g., avoid duplicate efforts) and promotes continuity of care.

Shift Reports

Shift reports are one of the most common forms of intraprofessional communication. Nurses have described barriers and facilitators during hand-off communication (Welsh, Flanagan, & Ebright, 2010). The nurses who were interviewed in the Welsh et al. study identified six such barriers: (1) too little information, (2) too much information, (3) inconsistent quality, (4) limited opportunity to ask questions, (5) equipment malfunction (e.g., tape recorders), and (6) interruptions. They also described some of the practical challenges (e.g., not having time to ask questions) during such hand-offs and noted how reports may vary by individual nurses. In addition, the nurses described four facilitators of hand-off communication: (1) "pertinent" content, (2) notes and space for notes, (3) face-to-face interactions with the outgoing nurse, and (4) structured form/checklists. Interestingly, they identified structured processes (e.g., face-to-face interactions) as important strategies to promote better communication.

Other researchers have described shift report as a highly interactive and time-intensive process in which nurses tailored their reports based on whether the oncoming nurse was familiar with the patient (Staggers & Jennings, 2009). They also described the content of a shift report as including facts as well as the nurse's clinical judgment, patient preferences, and recognition of the teamwork. Both studies identified interruptions as a barrier and structured formats as a way to facilitate effective communication (Staggers & Jennings, 2009: Welsh et al., 2010).

Transfer Reports

Transfers occur between units in the same institution or between different institutions. Intrahospital transfer communication issues have been found to vary by patient population (e.g., surgical patients) and type of transfer (e.g., Emergency Department) (Ong & Coiera, 2011). Within-hospital transfers often include both verbal and written communication between nurses. The verbal and written portions should complement each other and emphasize key issues, clinical findings, and anticipated care. However, nurses rarely talk with each other when a patient is transferred to another organization. In such instances, it is essential that nurses include critical information on the transfer form. So what can nurses do?

Ensuring Effective Intraprofessional Communication

Effective nurse–nurse handoffs entail at least two components: (1) clear communication of relevant information and (2) use of a structured approach to giving and receiving information.

First, nurses need to identify the relevant content, which will vary by the specific clinical unit, individual patient condition, and nurses' expertise and familiarity with the patient. Based on his or her clinical judgment, the nurse providing information should identify (1) obvious clinical priorities, (2) concerns requiring monitoring for early signs or symptoms of complications, (3) pending information that requires nursing action, and (4) information about ineffective and/or effective interventions. In the situation of a shift report, the oncoming nurse should be proactive in obtaining this essential information. Newly licensed nurses should ask more questions about unfamiliar information, terminology, or abbreviations. In the situation of a transfer, the receiving nurse should carefully read the referral information and if needed, contact the referring institution if information is missing or requires clarification.

Second, structured formats to give and/or document shift or transfer reports are being used to improve the consistency and quality of nurse-nurse communication. The Agency for Healthcare Research and Quality advocates several structured tools to improve communication among professionals, which were first developed by the Department of Defense's Patient Safety Program and in collaboration with them (AHRQ, 2013b). For example, the SBAR and I PASS the BATON mnemonics are two tools available on the AHRQ website.* The SBAR—Situation, Background, Assessment, Recommendations—format helps healthcare professionals when communicating with one another. By following this structure, nurses communicate the most relevant information and make recommendations for action that fosters collaboration among professionals. A modified SBAR format was advocated for use during bedside shift report that included patients and families (Baker, 2010). The author described the benefits of including patients in the process so they hear the exchange, can ask questions, and perhaps decrease their anxieties and promote their trust. Other nurses used the I PASS the BATON mnemonic (Table 18-1) for bedside shift report (Thomas & Donohue-Porter, 2011). Nurses were initially dissatisfied with the shift report process, but one of the benefits for newly licensed nurses was its use as a way to

---

*TeamSTEPPS® (http://teamstepps.ahrq.gov/) was developed by the Department of Defense's Patient Safety Program in collaboration with the Agency for Healthcare Quality and Research (Agency for Healthcare Quality and Research [AHRQ], 2013a; AHRQ, 2013b).

Table 18-1 I PASS the BATON Mnemonic

Step	Description
Introduction	Introduce yourself and your role/job (include the patient).
Patient	Identifiers, age, sex, location.
Assessment	Present chief complaint, vital signs, symptoms, and diagnosis.
Situation	Current status/circumstances, including code status, level of uncertainty, recent changes, and response to treatment.
Safety	Critical lab values/reports, socioeconomic factors, allergies, and alerts (e.g., falls, isolation).
THE	
Background	Comorbidities, previous episodes, current medications, and family history.
Actions	Which actions were taken or are required? Provide a brief rationale.
Timing	Level of urgency and explicit timing and prioritization of actions.
Ownership	Who is responsible (nurse/doctor/team)? Include patient/family responsibilities.
Next	What will happen next? Anticipated changes? What is the plan? Are there contingency plans?

Source: Agency for Healthcare Research and Quality. (2013b). TeamSTEPPS® fundamentals course: Module 6—Communication. http://www.ahrq.gov/teamsteppstools/instructor/fundamentals/module6/igcommunication.htm

know which information is included. In addition, the nurses took advantage of this tool as a time to teach and verify patient assessments, if needed.

In sum, nurses are expected to follow communication practices that minimize risks associated with hand-offs among providers and across transitions in care. One important initiative to help nurses develop these communication and teamwork competencies was begun by Quality and Safety Education for Nurses (QSEN, 2013), which has delineated specific knowledge, skill, and attitude statements for achieving competency in teamwork and collaboration for all prelicensure nurses entering practice. These competency statements summarize the salient points of this chapter (Table 18-2).

Table 18-2 Teamwork and Collaboration

Definition: Function effectively within nursing and interprofessional teams, fostering open communication, mutual respect, and shared decision making to achieve quality patient care.		
Knowledge	Skills	Attitudes
Describe own strengths, limitations, and values in functioning as a member of a team.	Demonstrate awareness of own strengths and limitations as a team member. Initiate plan for self-development as a team member. Act with integrity, consistency and respect for differing views.	Acknowledge own potential to contribute to effective team functioning. Appreciate importance of intraprofessional and interprofessional collaboration.
Describe scopes of practice and roles of healthcare team members. Describe strategies for identifying and managing overlaps in team member roles and accountabilities. Recognize contributions of other individuals and groups in helping patient/family achieve health goals.	Function competently within own scope of practice as a member of the healthcare team. Assume role of team member or leader based on the situation. Initiate requests for help when appropriate to situation. Clarify roles and accountabilities under conditions of potential overlap in team member functioning. Integrate the contributions of others who play a role in helping the patient/family achieve health goals.	Value the perspectives and expertise of all health team members. Respect the centrality of the patient/family as core members of any healthcare team. Respect the unique attributes that members bring to a team, including variations in professional orientations and accountabilities.

Knowledge	Skills	Attitudes
Analyze differences in communication style preferences among patients and families, nurses, and other members of the health team. Describe the impact of one's own communication style on others. Discuss effective strategies for communicating and resolving conflict.	Communicate with team members, adapting one's own style of communicating to the needs of the team and situation. Demonstrate commitment to team goals. Solicit input from other team members to improve individual, as well as team, performance. Initiate actions to resolve conflict.	Value teamwork and the relationships upon which it is based. Value different styles of communication used by patients, families, and healthcare providers. Contribute to resolution of conflict and disagreement.
Describe examples of the impact of team functioning on safety and quality of care. Explain how authority gradients influence teamwork and patient safety.	Follow communication practices that minimize risks associated with hand-offs among providers and across transitions in care. Assert own position/perspective in discussions about patient care. Choose communication styles that diminish the risks associated with authority gradients among team members.	Appreciate the risks associated with hand-offs among providers and across transitions in care.
Identify system barriers and facilitators of effective team functioning. Examine strategies for improving systems to support team functioning.	Participate in designing systems that support effective teamwork.	Value the influence of system solutions in achieving effective

Source: Cronenwett, L., et al. (2007). Quality and safety education for nurses. Nursing Outlook. Mosby. Reprinted with permission.

Summary

Interprofessional and intraprofessional communication processes pose special challenges for nurses. When communication strategies previously learned—specifically, the Two-Challenge Rule and CUS (see the *Delegation and Assertive Communication* chapter) are not effective in resolving conflict the nurse can make use of the DESC script. Today's healthcare practitioners working on interprofessional teams are expected to share a common set of core competencies for interprofessional collaborative practice. The four domains of learning for all team members include communication, teamwork, roles and responsibilities, and values and ethics. High-functioning teams also expect members to give one another constructive feedback and respectfully receive constructive criticism from others. The QSEN competency for teamwork and collaboration provides guiding statements describing requisite knowledge, skills, and attitudes for nurses entering practice. Gaining competence begins with self-awareness and requires ongoing practice and reflection, particularly after disquieting exchanges with team members. Questions for reflection include: What went well? What went poorly? What could I have done differently? Nurses are advised to turn challenging conversations into learning opportunities. Assisting all team members to learn, practice, and reflect upon shared interactions can be empowering experiences. Utilizing effective communication with team members, particularly in times of conflict and disagreement, may help reduce errors, improve patient care outcomes and team functioning, and lead to healthier relationship building. Further research is needed to examine the following issues:

- What is the impact of effective communication strategies on patient outcomes and medical errors?
- What is the impact of effective communication strategies on nurse and physician job satisfaction, and how does provider satisfaction relate to patient outcomes?
- How can ongoing communication skills training for practicing physicians and nurses and other healthcare team members have a career-long impact on their communication skills?

Case Study Resolution

The nurse chose to remain civil, calm, and focused when facing the resident's hostile behavior. The nurse de-escalated the conflict, thereby taking the focus away from a possible power struggle with the resident, while bringing the focus back to the patient. Rather than acting angrily or feeling intimidated, and thus avoiding a confrontation, the nurse understood how important it was to speak up to express a concern about patient safety. Having all salient information at hand, the nurse practiced the DESC script:

D: The charge nurse used SBAR to report the new patient finding of shortness of breath when starting the IV antibiotic. The nurse provided additional information that the nurse had previously neglected—that despite placing the patient on a 50% O_2 face mask, Mrs. T.'s O_2 saturation rate was now 89% with a respiratory rate of 30 bpm. (**D**escribed the specific situation or behavior and provided concrete evidence or data)

E: The nurse expressed the concern that the patient's shortness of breath appeared to worsen when the IV antibiotic was hung and that this reaction made her uncomfortable. The nurse informed the resident of her concern about a possible unknown allergic reaction and worsening respiratory status. (**E**xpressed how the situation makes you feel and what your concerns are)

S: The nurse suggested that the IV antibiotic be stopped until the resident could evaluate the patient. Because the nurse had neglected to introduce herself to the resident earlier during the phone call, she informed the resident that this was the first time she had cared for this patient; the resident, in turn, informed the nurse that she, too, was unfamiliar with this patient. Given the additional data, the resident agreed to evaluate the patient within the next half hour. (**S**uggested other alternatives and sought agreement)

C: The nurse agreed and also informed the resident that if the patient's condition worsened before the resident arrived, then the rapid response team would be called. The resident concurred. (**C**onsequences should be stated in terms of impact on established team goals or patient safety)

The nurse resisted intimidation by using a structured communication strategy. Without feeling intimidated, the nurse was not pressured to continue administering the medication and thus avoided a potential allergic reaction to the medication by the patient, which would have further compounded her compromised respiratory status. If the conflict resolution strategy chosen had not been effective, then the charge nurse would have recognized the need to call the supervisor for support. The nurse would report the resident's disruptive behavior, understanding that unresolved disruptive behaviors and incivility by team members threaten patient safety.

Evidence-Based Website

Safecoms.org. (2007). Patient safety through teamwork and communication. Retrieved from http://www.safecoms.org/

The Denver Health Medical Center was awarded an AHRQ Partnerships in Implementing Patient Safety (PIPS) grant for a project titled *Improving Patient Safety Through Provider Communication Strategy Enhancements*. The purpose of this project was to implement and evaluate a comprehensive team communication strategy, develop an implementation toolkit that could be generalized to other settings of care, and improve patient safety by decreasing errors related to team communication failures in the hospital setting. Expected project outcomes included the following:

- Decreased communication failures as a contributing factor in Patient Safety Net reports
- Decreased time to treatment for nonemergent patient care requiring consultation between physicians and nurses
- Improvement in a culture of patient safety
- Development of a toolkit that was to be generalized to other settings of care

The Hospital Survey on Patient Safety Culture (HSOPSC) was a survey that was administered prior to interventions to gather baseline data and post implementation to determine any changes from baseline in the staff perceptions of patient safety culture of the study units. The HSOPSC measured several safety dimensions, including frequency of event reporting, overall perceptions of safety, supervisor/manager expectations and actions promoting safety, organizational learning (continuous improvement), teamwork within hospital units, communication openness, feedback and communication about error, nonpunitive response to error, staffing, hospital management support for patient safety, teamwork across hospital units, and hospital hand-offs and transitions. The evaluation and analysis tools, an implementation toolkit, and additional resources can be found at the following website: http://www.safecoms.org/.

References

Agency for Healthcare Research and Quality. (2013a). TeamSTEPPS® fundamentals course: Module 5—Mutual support. Retrieved from http://www.ahrq.gov/teamsteppstools/instructor/fundamentals/module5/igmutualsupp.htm

Agency for Healthcare Research and Quality. (2013b). TeamSTEPPS® fundamentals course: Module 6—Communication. Retrieved from http://www.ahrq.gov/teamsteppstools/instructor/fundamentals/module6/igcommunication.htm

Baker, S. J. (2010). Bedside shift report improves patient safety and nurse accountability. *Journal of Emergency Nursing, 36,* 355–358.

Dingley, C., Daugherty, K., Derieg, M., & Persing, R. (2008). Improving patient safety through provider communication strategy enhancements. *Advances in Patient Safety: New Directions and Alternative Approaches—HRQ, 3,* 1–18.

Institute of Medicine. (2011). *The future of nursing: Leading change, advancing health.* Washington, DC: National Academies Press.

Institute for Safe Medication Practices. (2004). Intimidation: Practitioners speak up about this unresolved problem (Part I). ISMP Medication Safety Alerts. Retrieved from http://www.ismp.org/newsletters/acutecare/articles/20040311_2.asp

Interprofessional Education Collaborative Expert Panel. (2011). *Core competencies for interprofessional collaborative practice: Report of an expert panel.* Washington, DC: Author.

Larrabee, J. H., Janney, M. A., Ostrow, C. L., Withrow, M. L., Hobbs, G. R., & Burant, C. J. (2003). Predicting registered nurse job satisfaction and intent to leave. *Nursing Administration, 33*(5), 271–283.

Ong, M. S,., & Coiera, E. (2011). A systematic review of failures in handoff communication during intrahospital transfers. *Joint Commission Journal on Quality and Patient Safety, 37*(6), 274–284.

Quality and Safety Education for Nurses. (2013). Competencies, pre-licensure KSAs: teamwork and collaboration. Retrieved from http://qsen.org/competencies/pre-licensure-ksas/#teamwork_collaboration

Staggers, N., & Jennings, B. M. (2009). The content and context of shift report on medical and surgical units. *Journal of Nursing Administration, 39*(9), 393–398.

Thomas, L., & Donohue-Porter, P. (2011). Blending evidence and innovation: Improving intershift handoffs in a multihospital setting. *Journal of Nursing Care Quality, 27*(2), 116–124.

Welsh, C. A., Flanagan, M. E., & Ebright, P. (2010). Barriers and facilitators to nursing handoffs: Recommendations for redesign. *Nursing Outlook, 58*(3), 148–154.

CHAPTER NINETEEN

Electronic Communication: Media, Social Networking, Medical Records, and Email

Sheryl LaCoursiere, PhD, FNP-BC, APRN

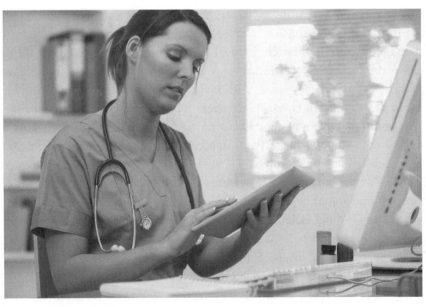

© Wavebreak Media/Thinkstock

■ CASE STUDY

Mary B. has been working in pediatric nursing in her regional specialty hospital for the past 10 years. She would like to do something more to help the parents who arrive with children with chronic medical problems but does not know where to start. Mary sees a wide range of problems and also sees that the parents of these patients bond with one another even when their children have different diagnoses. She sees that many of them are adept with the Internet. She knows that many parents exchange email addresses and "friend" each other on Facebook. She begins to consider which type of social networking venues might be the best avenues for these types of parents to communicate. She narrows down her search to Facebook and Twitter. She does look at LinkedIn but realizes it is more suited to professional social networking. Mary then decides to talk to several of these parents to see which parts of social networking they find most useful, and why, before she recommends anything further.

Introduction

Electronic communication comes in many forms. With the advent of increased bandwidth on the Internet and the proliferation of smartphones, electronic communication offers an instantaneous ability to relate to others. Types of media used for these exchanges now include traditional desktop computers as well as laptops; most recently, tablets have offered a portable alternative. At the same time, smartphones have been increasing in functionality, and the proliferation of applications ("apps") has enabled tracking of many phenomena, allowing one to view what information is "new" no matter where the user is logging in from. In addition, different types of apps have allowed for interchange of information from one type of media to another. For instance, a webpage accessed on a smartphone can be emailed and picked up on a desktop computer, from which it can then be printed. Many companies have websites as well as apps, with mechanisms that enable information to be exchanged between them. The ability to understand and teach patients to use social networking can have positive consequences, particularly in reaching patients in rural and underserved areas (Shaw & Johnson, 2011). The ability to use such media also has implications for our electronic communication with each other, as discussed in this chapter.

Social media refers to media that support electronic communication with other users. This communication may be synchronous, where the receiver is waiting and responding on the other end, or asynchronous, where communication may happen at any time, at each participant's convenience. In some cases, it may be a blend of the two. For instance, text messaging on a cell phone can be synchronous, when two parties are both present. It can also be used asynchronously, when one of the recipients may not see a message until a later time. As the use of cell phones has grown more ubiquitous, so has the use of messaging applications. These can range from basic text on simple cell phones in developing countries to the use of multicolor text and graphics on smartphones in more developed areas.

Social Networking

Social networking refers to communicating electronically using various types of social media. Social networking allows users to interchange ideas with each other, thereby enjoying the benefit of instantaneous communication and decreasing the users' isolation from one another. Social networking can involve contacting family and friends who are known to the sender, meeting new people through intermediaries, and reaching out and approaching persons previously unknown.

A disadvantage of social networking is the inability to see facial expressions and cues that are present in everyday face-to-face ("F2F") communication. As when email is used alone, users are left to interpret the meaning of ambiguous sentences. Was the sender angry or joking? Sometimes symbols such as emoticons provide cues—for instance, a "smiley face" ☺ indicates a positive meaning, and a frown a negative one ☹. Some venues for electronic communication, such as Skype (an alternative phone service), can lessen some of these misinterpretations by offering webcam capability, so the sender's face can be seen. Although this system is better than having no nonverbal cues at all, it can also be manipulated in that the recipient will see only the part of the sender that is in front of the camera.

In this chapter, we first discuss social networking applications in general for personal use and for use by patients and families; we then discuss professional use of social media.

Personal, Patient, and Family Social Networking

For general use, Facebook is a very good option for social networking, as well as discussion boards, Twitter, and Skype. We will go through each option in turn.

Facebook

Facebook allows users to connect with each other and be "friends." An account holder can post on his or her "wall," and others can read and respond to these postings. Communities or groups can be created around common interests. In either case, privacy can be restricted to those who are direct contacts or, conversely, settings can be made less restrictive so than anyone can read postings. Facebook allows users to form groups, which can be created to share common interests or support around a certain topic—for instance, Crohn's disease. Groups of a personal nature tend to be "closed." This means that potential members must be vetted by group leaders, and postings are not visible to casual Facebook readers.

Nurses can guide their patients to look for groups about health challenges they are facing. Caregivers can also create Facebook "pages" and start their own groups to update interested relatives and friends about the care of a particular patient.

Discussion Boards

Discussion boards are areas on websites where persons can "talk" to one another by means of "threads." Through this mechanism, one person will start a conversation, and others will follow, allowing a thread to be created. A new person coming in will see the flow of conversation between the previous parties.

Many discussion boards on the Internet have been established for support of various health and medical topics. The best way to find the most appropriate ones is to use a search engine with the wanted topic followed by "discussion boards." Another method to find relevant discussion boards is to visit the websites for the health problem in question—for instance, the American Diabetes Association operates discussion boards for persons with diabetes. Some discussion boards have fixed topics, but those that allow patients to determine their own concerns result in more postings (LaCoursiere, 2003).

Twitter

Twitter differs from Facebook in that one can "follow" anyone else without that person necessarily following the user back—unless the individual wants to. The Twitter user creates an account and has the ability to send out short messages ("tweets"), which must be less than 140 characters. Tweets can be directed to the world in general, or to specific tweeters. Over time, if a user tweets items that draw significant interest, the user will gain followers who find the tweets by searching for keywords. From a healthcare point of view, if the user was interested in heart disease, for example, he or she could follow the American Heart Association and receive breaking news. Some organizations pride themselves on tweeting at conferences, thereby ensuring that the general public will know what is going on inside, and followers will be among the first people to be apprised of new developments (McCartney, 2012).

A hashtag (#) with a particular name is added to each tweet for a particular event, so that others will be able to view all the tweets. For instance, a hashtag of #nurs2013 might be the tag for a nursing conference in 2013.

For those who are serious about tweeting, free software called TweetDeck allows a user to follow a number of keywords at once. Such software can also be very useful to communicate and receive news during emergencies and weather-related disasters.

Blogs

Blogs are online journals created by users, which others then read and respond to. Blogs can be found on many topics and health-related conditions. The nurse would want to be able to help patients and families find blogs on their conditions, bearing in mind that any advice therein would not take the place of advice from their healthcare provider. However, blogs can frequently offer a glimpse into the experience of someone else with the same condition.

Skype

Skype is an Internet version of a telephone that can also be used for social networking. Calls can be made internationally for free, with or without a webcam. A directory can be used to find people with similar interests for social networking purposes. Skype has an international flavor to it and displays the countries in which users are located. Thus, if a user was looking for contacts in Mexico, for instance, a directory search would be able to accommodate the search.

This is by no means an exclusive list of social networking sites. Many sites blur the boundaries between the various types of social media. For instance, they may seek to connect others with similar interests, such as a specific nationality or ethnic identity, but also simultaneously provide other content.

Professional Social Networking

To review professional social networking, we will first use the example of Facebook, and then LinkedIn. Both are available to be accessed on the Internet and also as apps for smartphones.

Facebook

In addition to the features listed earlier, for professional purposes there are a number of nursing resources available on Facebook. Many nursing organizations, such as the American Nurses Association, have a presence on Facebook. A nurse wanting to communicate with an organization or a particular specialty, for example, can do so on that entity's Facebook wall, as well as start a conversation with other nurses who have posted there. In addition, groups have been formed for nurses in certain regions of the country. Nurses returning to school—for instance, for an advanced practice degree—are also well represented. Nurses in these groups tend to compare notes on which schools have which requirements and how others are faring in going through their programs.

LinkedIn

LinkedIn is a professional social networking site that deserves special attention. The premise of LinkedIn is that it enables an individual to "connect" to people that the user knows; by accepting the user, these people let him or her into their network. Once inside a network, the individual is able to see the other user's connections. If the new user sees someone that he or she would like to know, the individual can ask the new connection to introduce them. LinkedIn also has plentiful discussion groups, some of which require the permission of the group leader to join. There are groups for many types of professional interests, as well as the ability to follow certain companies.

LinkedIn's internal search engine is very powerful, so that a user can search for potential contacts by location, industry, and school. For example, a person who wants to identify alumni of a particular school who live within 100 miles and work in the healthcare industry will be given a list sorted by users who are already contacts (first-degree connections), followed by those who are connected to someone in common (second-degree connections), and then those who are contacts of contacts—that is, two steps away (third-degree connections). As is the case with Facebook, users can allow built-in programs to go through their email inbox and find contacts who also use this social networking program.

Blogs

Many health professionals blog. An important point when using blogs for professional purposes is making sure that you do not violate any patient's privacy and confidentiality. For instance, if enough details are provided in a blog and the facility is small enough, the 56-year-old male patient who came in with a particular diagnosis and received care today might be able to be identified. If sufficient detail was made available, the patient or family member who saw this posting (even years later) might recognize themselves and initiate a lawsuit (Spector & Kappel, 2012).

Social networking can be used for personal as well as professional reasons. It allows connection with others who we may not see on a daily basis. A very important point is that information found on the Internet, although personal, may come to the attention of someone in a professional position; that individual might then use this information to evaluate a person, even if the information is from a personal account. For instance, a user may allow his or her postings to be viewed on Facebook by "friends of friends" only—but if one friend replies to a user's post, it may in turn be visible to that person's friends of friends, and so on. Large employers may assign human resources staffers to check Facebook pages of employees to see what is visible; if the information made available violates the organization's norms, it could present trouble for the user. In some cases, employers have asked potential employees to open their Facebook pages in their presence or asked for their passwords, although this practice has become illegal in some venues.

Most types of social networking have "push" and "pull" aspects to them. Teaser information is "pushed" to the user by email—for instance, which Facebook friends have updated their status, making the user curious to click and find out what the update is. For other less complex systems, such as discussion boards, the user may need to "pull" the information, or go in and read it without being prompted.

Thus there are both advantages and disadvantages to the use of social networking for personal and professional reasons. The nurse must be cognizant at every step of the potential implications of his or her actions. Because many social networking sites archive their material, a picture taken at a party while holding a glass of beer as a student may come back to haunt someone 5 years later when he or she is being evaluated for a promotion to nurse manager. The nurse must also keep in mind that many social networking sites are known for changing their rules and privacy settings with little warning, frequently using opt-out tactics. For instance, information that was previously not visible may now be opened up to "everyone," unless the user goes back in and adjusts a particular setting. If the user happens to not log in for several days, this change could be missed, and information that was thought to be private might now be visible to unwanted persons. There is also a professional responsibility to mentor the next generation and be sure that student nurses are adequately indoctrinated into the potential implications of social networking.

Medical Records

A discussion of electronic communication would not be complete without mentioning medical records. Whether these data are termed electronic health records (EHRs), which are more all-encompassing, or electronic medical records (EMRs), which record primarily medical information, the adoption of EHRs/EMRs means that the use of pure paper for health communication is diminishing. A large driver of this phenomenon is the U.S. government, which is beginning to offer reduced reimbursements for Medicare patients for facilities and practices that do not have their records in an electronic format. EHRs were initially developed for the hospital environment. However, as technology has evolved, EHRs have been adopted by many clinics as well as in long-term, rehabilitation, and home care settings. In addition, EHRs have been developed for specialty applications, such as neurology and psychiatry.

A major advantage of EHRs over paper records is the ability to review prior visits easily and detect trends in health status, whether it be narrative notes, vital signs, or lab values. With recent changes in health care, many smaller facilities are being purchased by larger networks, which presents challenges in terms of integrating different sets of records.

Email

Many EHR systems also have electronic communication built into them, allowing providers to communicate with one another as part of administering an individual patient's care. Although this would not be considered "social networking," it would fall under the realm of electronic health communication.

Several issues arise when considering email communication either within or outside of EHR systems. If the email is about or to and from a patient, care must be taken to make sure that the email is secure, whether it comprises a provider-to-provider or provider-to-patient message. A disclaimer focusing on confidentiality and privacy laws warns the recipient of potential ramifications of the email falling into the wrong hands.

In addition to understanding the legal ramifications, a healthcare agency must make decisions and establish policies regarding the use of email. Just as when users are visiting websites, email is void of the face-to-face contact that is so important in making clinical assessments. Although subjective data may be obtained, objective data are lost. Provider time must also be factored in, in terms of responding to and otherwise following up with email.

Conclusions

Nurses must also be cognizant to not relay any personally identifiable information via social media (Lyons & Reinisch, 2013). Official or unofficial rules regarding appropriate use of social media may be unintentionally violated, but there are still legal consequences (Spector & Kappel, 2012). In addition, because Internet access is not restricted to just the United States, an international perspective must be considered (Barry & Hardiker, 2012). Electronic communication technologies have the potential to advance patient–provider communication but must be used very carefully (Weaver, Lindsay, & Gitelman, 2012).

Summary

Electronic communication is an evolving phenomenon. Many electronic media are available through which to communicate, and many programs are offered in more than one format. Social networking has been growing exponentially, and frequently users have more than one option to access a particular program. Social networking offers a good way for patients to receive support; likewise, it enables nurses not only to communicate with one another, but also to serve as navigators in helping patients. Nurses must pay attention to evolving communication options via medical records and their resultant legal implications.

Case Study Resolution

Mary talks to several parents, who agree that they have found Facebook to be the best way to keep other family members and family friends updated on their child's condition. Many parents have started a special "page" devoted to their child. This has the advantage of keeping the information separate from their main Facebook page, and anyone wanting updates has to specifically subscribe to the child-focused page. This strategy ensures that casual acquaintances cannot see the details of the child's care the way a family member would. The page also keeps track of who has read it, so the parents can determine who has seen the most current updates. Parents also give the link to this page to other parents who they have met during their frequent office visits and hospitalizations. As a secondary source, they use Twitter for more general updates, especially on days when they are at the hospital and waiting for an appointment or procedure.

Websites

Allnurses.com

Allnurses.com is a social networking site for nurses that contains forums for nursing specialties and various levels of practice.

http://www.allnurses.com

American Nurses Association: *6 Tips for Nurses for Nurses Using Social Media*

The American Nurses Association provides tips for nurses using social media.

http://www.nursingworld.org/FunctionalMenuCategories/AboutANA/Social-Media/Social-Networking-Principles-Toolkit/Tip-Card-for-Nurses-Using-Social-Media.pdf (Pocket Card)

http://www.nursingworld.org/FunctionalMenuCategories/AboutANA/Social-Media/Social-Networking-Principles-Toolkit/6-Tips-for-Nurses-Using-Social-Media-Poster.pdf (Poster)

American Nurses Association: *Fact Sheet: Navigating the World of Social Media*

The American Nurses Association provides guidance for navigating social media.

http://www.nursingworld.org/FunctionalMenuCategories/AboutANA/Social-Media/Social-Networking-Principles-Toolkit/Fact-Sheet-Navigating-the-World-of-Social-Media.pdf

American Nurses Association: *Social Networking Principles Toolkit*

The American Nurses Association toolkit of social networking principles.

http://www.nursingworld.org/FunctionalMenuCategories/AboutANA/Social-Media/Social-Networking-Principles-Toolkit.aspx

Facebook

Social networking site.

http://www.facebook.com

National Council of State Boards of Nursing: *Social Media Guidelines*

The National Council of State Boards of Nursing provides social media guidelines.

https://www.ncsbn.org/2930.htm

National Council of State Boards of Nursing: *White Paper: A Nurse's Guide to the Use of Social Media*

The National Council of State Boards of Nursing white paper on the use of social media.

https://www.ncsbn.org/Social_media_guidelines.pdf

National Council of State Boards of Nursing: *ANA and NCSBN Unite to Provide Guidelines on Social Media and Networking for Nurses*

The National Council of State Boards of Nursing discussions with the American Nurses Association on social media.

https://www.ncsbn.org/2927.htm

LinkedIn

Professional social networking site.

http://www.linkedin.com

Skype

An alternative phone service where users may connect via the Internet and use web cameras to see one another.

http://www.skype.com

Twitter

A social networking program where users send out 140-character messages called tweets.

http://www.twitter.com

References

Barry, J., & Hardiker, N. R. (2012). Advancing nursing practice through social media: A global perspective. *Online Journal of Issues in Nursing, 17*(3), 5.

LaCoursiere, S. P. (2003). Telehealth support in cardiovascular disease. National Technical Information Service Report # PB2006-107544. Retrieved from http://www.ntis.gov/search/product.aspx?ABBR=PB2006107544

Lyons, R., & Reinisch C. (2013). The legal and ethical implications of social media in the emergency department. *Advanced Emergency Nursing Journal, 35*, 53–56. doi: 10.1097/TME.0b013e31827a4926

McCartney, P. (2012). Twitter at a nursing conference. *MCN American Journal of Maternal Child Nursing, 37*, 402. doi: 10.1097/NMC.0b013e31826ae034

Shaw, R. J., & Johnson, C. M. (2011). Health information seeking and social media use on the internet among people with diabetes. *Online Journal of Public Health Informatics, 3*(1), 3561.

Spector, N., & Kappel, D. M. (2012). Guidelines for using electronic and social media: The regulatory perspective. *Online Journal of Issues in Nursing, 17*(3), 1.

Weaver, B., Lindsay, B., & Gitelman. B. (2012). Communication technology and social media: Opportunities and implications for healthcare systems. *Online Journal of Issues in Nursing, 17*(3), 3.

Additional References

Fisher, J., & Clayton. M. (2012). Who gives a tweet: Assessing patients' interest in the use of social media for health care. *Worldviews on Evidence-Based Nursing, 9*, 100–198. doi: 10.1111/j.1741-6787.2012.00243.x

Jacobson, J. (2011). Leveling the research field through social media. *American Journal of Nursing, 111*(10), 14–15. doi: 10.1097/01.NAJ.0000406403.80894.94

McCartney, P. R. (2012). Social networking principles for nurses. *MCN American Journal of Maternal Child Nursing, 37*(2), 131. doi: 10.1097/NMC.0b013e3182430380

Pattillo, R. E. (2012). Who is in control of social networks? *Nurse Educator, 37*, 232. doi: 10.1097/NNE.0b013e31826f282b

Randolph, S. A. (2012). Using social media and networking in health care. *Workplace Health and Safety, 60*(1), 44. doi: 10.3928/21650799-20111227-14

Rice, M. J. (2013). Social media in healthcare: Educational policy implications. *Archives of Psychiatric Nursing, 27*, 61–62. doi: 10.1016/j.apnu.2012.11.001

Schuring, L. T. (2011). Social media: A communication responsibility. *ORL Head and Neck Nursing, 29*(3), 5–6.

CHAPTER TWENTY

Delegation and Assertive Communication

JoAnn Mulready-Shick

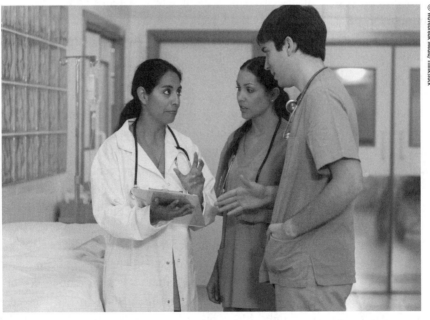

■ CASE STUDY

The newly licensed registered night nurse on a surgical unit received a report about a new patient, Mr. H. Mr. H. is an alert and oriented 78-year-old male, with a history of type 1 diabetes and sleep apnea treated by continuous positive airway pressure (CPAP), who just had eye surgery for a detached retina. After midnight, the patient complained of inadequate eye pain control despite administration of scheduled narcotics. After administering an additional narcotic dose, the nurse became concerned upon finding the patient lethargic and decided that more frequent assessments were needed. The nurse told the experienced nursing assistant to check on him in a half hour rather than the usual "every 4 hours" and report back any changes in the patient's condition. The nursing assistant replied, "Can't you see I am too busy? You will be lucky if I can get to him in an hour." The nurse, fearful of a confrontation, simply restated the request for the nursing assistant to obtain additional vital signs when able; then the nurse went on caring for another patient.

Introduction

How does the nurse in the case study communicate a sense of urgency for performing this delegated task and thus prevent a delay in care? How might the nurse approach this team member assertively and respectfully while keeping patient safety a priority? Communication challenges in contemporary nursing and health care abound. Given the increasing demand for nursing services in conjunction with a growing elder population, nurses often must rely heavily on team members, particularly unlicensed assistive nursing staff, to meet the complex healthcare needs of patients. In turn, communication practices while working with others have never been more important. Positive communication among members of the healthcare team supports the provision of safe, patient-centered care. Patients' preferences, values, and needs are best addressed when healthcare team members effectively communicate. Providing high-quality care, including effective communication among all team members, is challenging at best while often working amidst chaotic situations and ever-changing healthcare systems.

It is no wonder that communication failures among healthcare team members are reported to be at an all-time high. Poor communication among coworkers is commonly identified as a cause of nurse job dissatisfaction and viewed as a significant component of unhealthy work environments and malpractice claims

(Controlled Risk Insurance Company, 2013; Kupperschmidt, Kientz, Ward, & Reinholz, 2010). Communication errors among staff members have also been identified by The Joint Commission as a frequent root cause across all types of sentinel events.* In fact, communication error, in combination with human factors and leadership error, is recognized as the most common root cause of the majority of sentinel events (Joint Commission, 2011). Improving the effectiveness of communication among professional caregivers has been targeted as an important National Patient Safety Goal. Specifically, the reporting of critical results of tests and diagnostic procedures on a timely basis and maintaining and communicating accurate patient medication information were identified as recent goals by The Joint Commission (2013). Quality and safety go hand in hand with improving communication on healthcare teams. Therefore, promoting healthy communication among healthcare team members starts with building and utilizing teams who collaborate and communicate effectively.

Effective Communication Standards and Strategies

Effective communication can be promoted with the use of communication standards and strategies. These standards are a helpful guide for the nurse to follow when relaying patient care information to team members.

In the chapter-opening case study, how aware was the nurse of this interaction with the nursing assistant? How aware are you of the multiple messages conveyed to the myriad team members during one day at work?

All effective communication begins with self-awareness. The nurse can use the communication standards in Box 20-1 as a checklist in assessing his or her present competency level and in identifying strategies for improved communication with team members. The consequences of not communicating effectively are significant. Negative, inappropriate, or inadequate interactions between the nurse and another team member may impede the nurse's ability to obtain the collaboration necessary to carry out proper delegation for implementing safe patient care and lead to conflict, dissatisfaction among team members, and, eventually, poor patient outcomes.

---

*A sentinel event is an unexpected occurrence involving death or serious physical or psychological injury, or the risk thereof.

Box 20-1 Communication Standards

- Complete
- Communicates all relevant information
- Clear
- Conveys information that is plainly understood
- Brief
- Communicates the information in a concise manner
- Timely
- Offers and requests information in an appropriate timeframe
- Verifies authenticity
- Validates or acknowledges information

Source: Agency for Healthcare Research and Quality. (2013b). TeamSTEPPS® fundamentals course: Module 6—Communication. Retrieved from http://www.ahrq.gov/teamsteppstools/instructor/fundamentals/module6/igcommunication.htm

---

Self-awareness also includes recognizing common barriers to effective communication (Box 20-2). It is evident that a number of possible barriers may have occurred in the case study, such as lack of information sharing, hierarchy, defensiveness, lack of follow-up with a coworker, and excessive workload.

Communication Strategies: Check-Back, Call-Out, Two-Challenge Rule, and CUS

In addition to tackling communication barriers, nurses can improve communication and teamwork skills by utilizing common communication strategies. TeamSTEPPS® is an evidence-based teamwork system for clinical practice aimed at optimizing patient outcomes among all healthcare team members (TeamSTEPPS®, 2013).* In particular, two important communication strategies for improving communication and patient safety include Check-Back and Call-Out (AHRQ, 2013a & 2013b). When using Check-Back, three steps occur: (1) the

---

*TeamSTEPPS® (http://teamstepps.ahrq.gov/) was developed by the Department of Defense's Patient Safety Program in collaboration with the Agency for Healthcare Quality and Research (Agency for Healthcare Quality and Research [AHRQ], 2013a; AHRQ, 2013b).

| **Box 20-2** | Barriers to Effective Communication |

- Inconsistency in team membership
- Lack of time
- Lack of information sharing
- Hierarchy
- Defensiveness
- Conventional thinking
- Complacency
- Varying communication styles
- Conflict
- Lack of coordination
- Lack of follow-up with coworkers
- Distractions
- Fatigue
- Workload
- Misinterpretation of cues
- Lack of role clarity

Source: Agency for Healthcare Research and Quality. (2013b). TeamSTEPPS® fundamentals course: Module 6—Communication. Retrieved from http://www.ahrq.gov/teamsteppstools/instructor/fundamentals/module6/igcommunication.htm

sender initiates the messages, (2) the receiver accepts the message, and (3) the receiver provides feedback and confirmation. Checking back is an especially important strategy because clinical conversations happen quickly and healthcare providers can be distracted by numerous issues.

Another effective strategy for the nursing assistant, or any team member, to employ when encountering an emergency is Call-Out. Call-Out is used to communicate critical information to all team members during emergent or actual emergency situations, such as finding the patient without a pulse or respirations. Call-Out helps all members of the team to anticipate the next steps in care. Which information would the nursing assistant be expected to call out? In your daily nursing practice, which information would you want called out?

Nurses are expected to demonstrate effective communication skills in every interaction with team members by following a set of shared standards of communication and common communication strategies. One particular strategy that is helpful for everyday nursing practice is the use of assertive communication. Learning to communicate effectively and assertively does not often come naturally, but rather develops in tandem with learning new skills and after much practice (including role-playing) and reflection. In the case study, the nurse did not restate the concern or provide information to the nursing assistant about why this patient was a priority. Communication would have been improved if the nurse had used the following two approaches for speaking with assertiveness: the Two-Challenge Rule and the CUS (C = Concern, U = Uncomfortable, and S = Safety Issue) strategy.

The Two-Challenge Rule is particularly useful when the nurse encounters departures from standards of practice, unprofessional behaviors, or disregard of his or her initial assertion (AHRQ, 2013a). Had the nurse responded with this strategy, the nurse would have expressed the concern about the patient's change (e.g., increased lethargy) at least twice, first by forming a question and second by providing some supporting evidence for the concern (e.g., comparing the patient's responsiveness over time). The Two-Challenge Rule ensures that the communication exchange has been heard, understood, and acknowledged by the other party. In this case, the nursing assistant acknowledged the nurse's request, but the nurse failed to fully communicate its seriousness; in turn, the nursing assistant's response conveyed both a sense of being overwhelmed and the view that the delegated task was not a top priority.

A second approach, the CUS strategy, has also been found to be specifically effective in developing assertiveness when interacting with team members, peers, physicians, and nursing assistants (AHRQ, 2013b). CUS is a three-step process that can assist the nurse in stopping an activity or drawing attention to an interaction when the nurse senses a potential safety issue or discovers a break in safety. The CUS strategy provides the nurse with an effective approach for communicating with assertiveness and a clear focus. Let's think about how the nurse could have spoken with assertiveness with the nursing assistant in the case study by using the CUS strategy. The nurse might have stated:

> I am really Concerned about Mr. H. I am Uncomfortable that he has become increasingly lethargic in the past half hour. This is a Safety issue because I gave him additional pain medication for his eye pain, so

he needs closer monitoring right now. He needs vital signs taken more frequently. Please take his vital signs in a half-hour, also checking on how alert he is, and report back to me at that time.

When a team member uses the Two-Challenge Rule and the CUS strategy, all members immediately understand the focus of concern, its implications, and actions that need to be taken to address the situation. When teams regularly practice effective communication strategies, all team members become familiar with this process for opening up communication. In this case, the nursing assistant would have likely understood the importance of carrying out this patient care activity and shifted priorities, raised questions with the nurse, or requested assistance so Mr. H. would have received more frequent monitoring.

When speaking and using assertive communication strategies, the nurse begins statements with the word "I" rather than "you". Using "you" is often perceived as an aggressive message, communicating hostility, intimidation, or power over another and can lead to defensiveness and breaks in patient safety and quality. For example, note the nursing assistant's response to the nurse's request in the case study. In contrast, using "I" sends a message of direct, specific, and genuine concern while respecting the rights of others.

Using assertiveness first and foremost is important for providing safe, patient-centered care. Most nurses do not come readily prepared with such assertive communication skills. The nurse may shy away from acting assertively for fear of being seen as too aggressive or superior to others or to avoid potential conflict. Some nurses may have learned passive communication patterns from past personal experiences, from family, or as part of their cultural patterns. In contrast, other nurses may use an aggressive communication style in the workplace, having learned this style at home, from particular relationships, or from past work experiences. In this case, this nurse's or team member's communication exchanges would need to be toned down, and made less forceful, to ensure effective team interactions. A nurse should communicate neither passively nor aggressively, but rather assertively as a healthcare team member who develops and fulfills the nurse's role as patient advocate in promoting safe quality care.

Effective Delegation

Delegating effectively is a critical challenge for nurses today. Communication within healthcare teams involves not only effective and assertive communication skills, but also skill in distinguishing which aspects of patient care can be delegated and which cannot. Assertive and clear communication goes hand in hand with delegating patient care tasks to nursing assistants. In contemporary nursing practice across all settings, from home care, to long-term care, to acute care, nurses are delegating a wide range of patient care activities. The importance of effective team functioning and "working with and through others and the abilities to delegate, assign, manage and supervise have never been as critical and challenging as in the complex and complicated world of 21st century health care" (National Council of State Boards of Nursing [NCBSN]), 2005b, p. 3).

To determine how to safely and effectively delegate aspects of care to competent others, important principles are outlined by regulatory agencies, particularly the NCSBN. Delegation is defined as "the act of transferring to a competent individual the authority to perform a selected nursing task in a selected situation, and the process for doing the work" (NCSBN, 2005b, p. 1). The important documents published by the NCSBN provide guidance and outline key concepts and principles for the nurse in delegation decision making (Box 20-3 and Box 20-4).

Box 20-3 Delegation Key Concepts

- Delegation is a skill requiring clinical judgment and final accountability for client care.
- The steps of the delegation process include:
  1. Assessment of the client, the staff, and the context of the situation
  2. Communication to provide direction and opportunity for interaction during the completion of the delegated task
  3. Surveillance and monitoring to assure compliance with standards of practice, policies, and procedures
  4. Evaluation to consider the effectiveness of the delegation and whether the desired client outcome was attained
- Boards of nursing regulate nursing practice.
- Nurse practice acts determine which level of licensed nurse is authorized to delegate.
- Assessment, planning, evaluation, and nursing judgment cannot be delegated.

Source: National Council of State Boards of Nursing. (2005b). Working with others: A position paper. Retreived from https://www.ncsbn.org/Working_with_Others.pdf

| **Box 20-4** | Delegation Principles |

- The nurse may delegate components of care but does not delegate the nursing process itself.

- The decision of whether to delegate or assign is based upon the nurse's judgment concerning the condition of the patient, the competence of all members of the nursing team, and the degree of supervision that will be required of the nurse if a task is delegated.

- The nurse delegates only those tasks for which she or he believes the other health-care worker has the knowledge and skill to perform, taking into consideration training, cultural competence, experience, and facility/agency policies and procedures.

- The nurse individualizes communication regarding the delegation to the nursing assistive personnel and client situation, and the communication should be clear, concise, correct, and complete. The nurse verifies comprehension with the nursing assistive personnel and that the assistant accepts the delegation and the responsibility that accompanies it.

- Communication must be a two-way process. Nursing assistive personnel should have the opportunity to ask questions and/or for clarification of expectations.

- The nurse uses critical thinking and professional judgment when following the Five Rights of Delegation, to be sure that the delegation or assignment is:

  1. The right task

  2. Under the right circumstances

  3. To the right person

  4. With the right directions and communication

  5. Under the right supervision and evaluation.

Source: National Council of State Boards of Nursing. (2005a). ANA and NCSBN joint statement on delegation. Retrieved from https://www.ncsbn.org/Delegation_joint_statement_NCSBN-ANA.pdf

Nurses often verbalize discomfort with the delegation process and communication during delegation. Oftentimes, the nurse's discomfort in delegation situations stems from different sources depending on the situation. For example, nurses must be confident with their clinical judgment and the appropriateness of the activity to be delegated. Once the nurse recognizes the need for delegation, the nurse must clearly communicate the task being delegated along with any parameters, time frame, and follow-up. As discussed, the nurse must develop assertive communication skills, while recognizing that communication is a two-way process (Table 20-1).

Table 20-1 Communication Must Be a Two-Way Process

The Nurse	The Nursing Assistive Personnel	Documentation

• Assesses the assistant's understanding
 	
  • How the task is to be accomplished
 	
  • When and what information is to be reported, including:
 	
    • Expected observations to report and record
 	
    • Specific client concerns that would require prompt reporting
 	
• Individualizes for the nursing assistive personnel and client situation
 	
• Addresses any unique client requirements and characteristics and articulates clear expectations
 	
• Assesses the assistant's understanding of expectations, providing clarification if needed
 	
• Communicates his or her willingness and availability to guide and support the assistant
 	
• Assures appropriate accountability by verifying that the receiving person accepts the delegation and accompanying responsibility
	• Asks questions regarding delegation and seek clarification of expectations if needed
	
	• Informs the nurse if the assistant has not done a task/function/activity before, or has done it only infrequently
	
	• Asks for additional training or supervision
	
	• Affirms understanding of expectations
	
	• Determines the communication method between the nurse and the assistive personnel
	
	• Determines the communication and plan of action in emergency situations
		• Is timely, complete, and accurate documentation of provided care
		
		• Facilitates communication with other members of the healthcare team
		
		• Records the nursing care provided

Source: National Council of State Boards of Nursing. (2005a). ANA and NCSBN joint statement on delegation. Retrieved from https://www.ncsbn.org/Delegation_joint_statement_NCSBN-ANA.pdf

Summary

Communication processes are challenging for all nurses, but particularly for those who are new to the profession. To practice in and uphold a culture of quality and safety nurses must communicate effectively with all team members. Promoting healthy, assertive communication among healthcare team members starts with building and utilizing effective teamwork and with recognizing common barriers to effective communication. It is important for the nurse to use current standards and strategies for effective communication. Becoming competent in effective communication skills begins with a nurse's self-awareness and requires ongoing practice. Communication strategies that have been identified as promoting safer patient care and more effective interactions among team members include Check-Back, Call-Out, the Two-Challenge Rule, and the CUS strategy. Developing knowledge, skills, and attitudes that support delegating patient care is an essential competency for today's professional nurse. Communication during delegation can be enhanced with the use of assertive communication skills and guidelines provided by the NCSBN.

Case Study Resolution

Closer examination of the communication exchange in this patient care scenario points to needed improvements by both parties—the nurse *and* the nursing assistant. There were several problems with how the nurse delegated the task to the nursing assistant. Some of the major problems were the use of ambiguous language (i.e., "check on him") and failure to demonstrate assertive communication because of a fear of conflict compounded by a lack of experience. Specifically, the nurse did not communicate his or her concern with relevant data—that is, Mr. H.'s increased lethargy after the nurse had given him an additional dose of pain medication. As discussed in this chapter, the nurse could have used Check-Back, the Two-Challenge Rule, or the CUS strategy. Specifically, the "red flag" in this interaction was the nursing assistant's response, "Can't you see I am too busy? You'll be lucky if I can get to him in an hour," indicating a refusal to accept a legitimate, delegated activity. This response should have caught the nurse's attention and led to several immediate strategies to address the communication and the needed care for the patient. It was clear that the nursing assistant did not understand the urgency of the situation because the nurse did not provide meaningful information.

In this case study, the nurse was bothered by the nursing assistant's response, along with the suddenness of Mr. H.'s change in responsiveness, and feared confronting a team member. The nurse decided to talk with an experienced nurse on the unit. Together they reviewed the clinical situation and determined how to best delegate the task to the nursing assistant. After role-playing with the more experienced nurse, the nurse found the nursing assistant to discuss the situation. The nurse started the conversation: "I wanted to follow up because Mr. H. needs to be closely monitored, and I know you have a lot of other things to do. I'm really concerned with the change in Mr. H.'s lethargy since he received his pain medication. We need to do frequent vital signs every 15 minutes for the next hour. Will you be able to do that?" The nursing assistant reordered priorities and monitored Mr. H.'s vital signs, which stabilized. He became increasingly responsive with no further complaints of pain. The nursing assistant provided the nurse with the updated information as asked.

Evidence-Based Article

Anthony, M. K., & Vidal, K. (2010). Mindful communication: A novel approach to improving delegation and increasing patient safety. *Online Journal of Issues in Nursing, 15*(2), 1–13.

The article provides a rationale for the conceptual basis of the linkages among safety, information quality, mindful communication, and contextual influences. The authors' review of the literature suggests that delegation issues and the tasks that are delegated have not changed much over the years; however, the context and work environment in which these tasks occur have changed dramatically. They assert that challenges remain in providing the "right communication" during the delegation process. Further, they contend that the nature of the information between the nurse and assistive personnel is often not communicated in a timely way, or the meaning of the information is uncertain, leading to information not being passed on; the unintended consequences may include subsequent care being inappropriate, missed, or delayed, and ultimately poor patient outcomes. The authors recommend integrating a mindful communication practice, which recognizes the significance of the facts and illuminates how they pertain to the patient situation, as a principle of delegation. The implications relevant to this chapter are the importance of the nurse and nursing assistant having a trusting relationship, and the need for them to enter into shared mindful communication as a necessary condition for delegation, which can lead to a higher quality of work and improved patient outcomes.

References

Agency for Healthcare Research and Quality. (2013a). TeamSTEPPS® fundamentals course: Module 5—Mutual support. Retrieved from http://www.ahrq.gov/teamsteppstools/instructor/fundamentals/module5/igmutualsupp.htm

Agency for Healthcare Research and Quality. (2013b). TeamSTEPPS® fundamentals course: Module 6—Communication. Retrieved from http://www.ahrq.gov/teamsteppstools/instructor/fundamentals/module6/igcommunication.htm

Controlled Risk Insurance Company. 2013. Communication. Retrieved from http://www.rmf.harvard .edu/Clinician-Resources/Topic-Tag/Communication

Joint Commission. (2011). Sentinel event data. Root causes by event type: 2004–2012. Retrieved from http://www.jointcommission.org/assets/1/18/Root_Causes_Event_Type_04_4Q2012.pdf

Joint Commission. (2013). National patient safety goals. Retrieved from http://www.jointecommission.org/assets/1/18/NPSG_Chapter_Jan2013_HAP.pdf

Kupperschmidt, B., Kientz, E., Ward, J., & Reinholz, B. (2010). A healthy work environment: It begins with you. *Online Journal of Issues in Nursing, 15*(1), 1–10.

National Council of State Boards of Nursing. (2005a). ANA and NCSBN joint statement on delegation. Retrieved from https://www.ncsbn.org/Delegation_joint_statement_NCSBN-ANA.pdf

National Council of State Boards of Nursing. (2005b). Working with others: A position paper. Retrieved from https://www.ncsbn.org/Working_with_Others.pdf

TeamSTEPPS®. (2013). TeamSTEPPS®: Home. Retrieved from http://teamstepps.ahrq.gov/.

Conclusion

CHAPTER TWENTY-ONE

A Conclusion and a Beginning

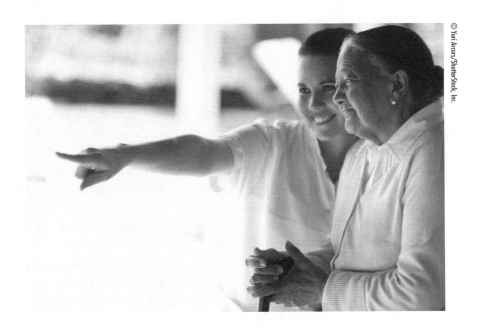

■ **CASE STUDY**

Theresa is a 72-year-old woman with non-small-cell lung cancer who has been treated with intravenous (IV) chemotherapy for more than a year. Today, she arrives in the ambulatory cancer center with Joe, her husband of 51 years. Over the last year of chemotherapy, Theresa has experienced numerous problems with IV access but remains good-natured and often makes jokes with the staff. She recently had her chest port removed because of thrombus formation. Theresa's remaining veins are small and very fragile, requiring the most experienced nurse, Tina, to start her IV. After Tina has two unsuccessful attempts, Theresa, in her good-natured way, says, "We had better call in the professionals." The "professionals" to whom she refers are the IV nurses at the hospital. Because the IV team is short staffed, it could be hours before Theresa would have her IV inserted and begin her day of chemotherapy.

The Nurse as a Communicator

The effectiveness of nursing care is strengthened by good communication skills. Patients often share their stories, symptoms, and concerns during routine care. Both the patients' spoken words and their nonverbal communication convey important information about their experiences and needs. Assessing and listening to patients provides valuable insights while nurses establish therapeutic relationships and trusting environments where they understand their patients and their patients, in turn, feel comfortable sharing information.

Effective nursing communication is very powerful. It can put a patient at ease, set up a productive relationship, enable more accurate assessment of patients' conditions and concerns, offer support, facilitate decision making, and deliver effective interventions. There is no other skill that is used more in nursing than communication. Nurses create open environments and treat patients with honesty and respect. They strive to understand patients' and families' concerns and needs so they can individualize their care plans.

While watching nursing students in the clinical setting, it became apparent that many students were unsure about how to talk with patients. Often, students focused on their skills sheet and tried to perfect their technical skills, such as performing intramuscular injections or dressing changes. However, before any technical intervention can take place, communication must begin between the nurse and the patient. Meeting a new postoperative patient at the start of a shift, assessing a woman in labor, educating a patient about diabetes, setting treatment goals with a patient with breast cancer—all of these encounters begin with communication. And good communication skills are not only important for relaying information: Nurses are also essential for establishing trust and rapport, showing respect for the needs and feelings of patients, and reaping the rewards of connecting with other people who are the recipients of nursing care.

Nurses enter their profession for different reasons. The most frequently cited reason is because nurses enjoy helping other people. Today, when encounters with patients are limited by time constraints and workloads, it is even more important to condense the important aspects of good communication. This text is not meant to simplify a skill that is never truly perfected, but rather explores some basic concepts about communication that can be taught in nursing school and refined over time. These beginning skills permit students to develop confidence in, and reflect on, their abilities to communicate, which in turn allows them to evolve their own communication style over years of nursing practice.

Nurses have a unique position within the healthcare system. They communicate with patients for extended periods of time, providing opportunities for disclosure by patients. Often personal revelations from patients occur spontaneously during routine care, such as while taking vital signs during the night. These moments may become times for providing support and comfort, away from the scheduled testing, interventions, and business of a healthcare facility. Such moments may also be some of the most rewarding in a nursing career because the nurse was trusted with these revelations and personal searches for meaning during a health crisis.

Nurses also communicate with other healthcare professionals—doctors, physical and occupational therapists, dieticians, and social workers, to name just a few. Nurses tend to be the "center" of communication between different departments and professions, advocating for patients and helping them navigate the healthcare system. They can use assertive communication and negotiation skills to advocate for patients as well as maintain their own personal integrity. In this way, communication in nursing is unique, making it crucial in achieving positive outcomes for patients.

No one ever masters communication skills. Nurses learn constantly from every patient encounter and when working both with families and with the healthcare team. With time and experience, they become flexible communicators, adapting their approach and style from room to room, bed to bed, and chair to chair. Because nursing communication is adaptable and respectful, each patient is approached as a unique human being. While not every encounter is satisfying or rewarding, less than exemplary experiences provide nurses with opportunities to learn about others and themselves.

Patients share so much of themselves with nurses. Sometimes it changes our perspectives, prompts a laugh, or forces us to rethink long-held notions about life and health care. But mostly, nurses are privileged to be part of patients' lives, permitted into very personal experiences, and then trusted to make a difference in their health and well-being. Good communication enhances the nurse–patient relationship, making a better healthcare experience for the patient and a more rewarding career for the nurse.

How nurses use their communication skills with patients evolves with time and experience and varies by clinical setting and situation. Nurses, like patients, have unique personalities that shape how they talk with patients. Some nurses have a gentle touch, a great sense of humor, a gift for counseling, an uncanny ability to understand their patients' needs, or quick assessment skills. Celebrating these individual gifts and using them to promote healing is what makes nursing such a rewarding career. Nursing provides a unique opportunity—the chance to communicate and connect with people to improve their health.

Case Study Resolution

Knowing that Theresa has a good sense of humor and trusts the nursing staff, Tina and the other oncology nurses decide to try one more time—but this time they use "special effects." Tina says, "Theresa, would you let us try one more time? We have one more trick up our sleeves. If this doesn't work, we will call in the professionals." The nurses turned the lights off and walked slowly across the room with the "vein finder," the two-pronged lighted device often used to find deep veins in pediatric patients. As they approach Theresa, the two dots of light from the device light the darkened room. The nurses make the sound of a drum roll. Theresa starts to laugh and concedes to one more try. This time, success! The IV line is in. As Tina and the other nurses thank her for her patience, Theresa says, "I think the professionals are here."

INDEX

Note: Page numbers followed by *b, f,* or *t* indicate material in boxes, figures, or tables, respectively.

A

acceptance, 187
acknowledgment (renewal stress), 209
active leadership role of nurses, 16
active listening, 80–82
  barriers to, 82–83
  body language evaluation, 99
  body posture during, 82
  during the outburst, 202
actual simulation case, 154
adaptation and change, 209
additive responses, 86
adolescents, communicating
    with, 145*t,* 147
adult stage of development, 19*t*
advance directives, 30, 191
Agency for Healthcare Research and
    Quality (AHRQ), 238
aggression, 204

allow natural death (AND), 192
altruism, 64, 222
American Diabetes Association, 250
American Heart Association, 251
American Hospital Association,
    "A Patient's Bill of Rights," 30
American Nurses Association (ANA), 28
  Code of Ethics for Nurses, 31, 34–35
  Social Policy Statement, 31
American Pain Society, 181
anger
  dealing with expressions of, 203*b*
  expressions of patient, 201–204
  during life-threatening illness, 187
  resolve the issues, 204
  response to, 201–204
  work through, 202
anticipatory grieving, 187
anticonvulsants, 177
antidepressants, 177